THE
VITAMIN
CURE
for Migraines

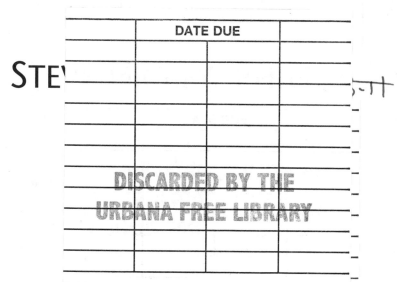
STE٬   ;-11

**Basic
Health**
PUBLICATIONS, INC.

The information contained in this book is based upon the research and personal and professional experiences of the author. It is not intended as a substitute for consulting with your physician or other healthcare provider. Any attempt to diagnose and treat an illness should be done under the direction of a healthcare professional.

The publisher does not advocate the use of any particular healthcare protocol but believes the information in this book should be available to the public. The publisher and author are not responsible for any adverse effects or consequences resulting from the use of the suggestions, preparations, or procedures discussed in this book. Should the reader have any questions concerning the appropriateness of any procedures or preparation mentioned, the author and the publisher strongly suggest consulting a professional healthcare advisor.

Basic Health Publications, Inc.
28812 Top of the World Drive
Laguna Beach, CA 92651
949-715-7327 • www.basichealthpub.com

Library of Congress Cataloging-in-Publication Data

Hickey, Steve
   The vitamin cure for migraines / Steve Hickey.
      p. cm.
   Includes bibliographical references and index.
   ISBN 978-1-59120-267-7
   1. Migraine. 2. Orthomolecular therapy. I. Title.
   RC392.H525   2010
   616.8'491206—dc22
                                                2009044167

Editor: John Anderson
Typesetting/Book design: Gary A. Rosenberg
Cover design: Mike Stromberg

Printed in the United States of America

10   9   8   7   6   5   4   3   2   1

CONTENTS

ACKNOWLEDGMENTS

An author producing a book on such a complex topic with a reasonable level of readability must rely on the help and support of others. This book depended on the expert assistance of Dr. Hilary Roberts, who read the manuscript, made suggestions, and corrected errors. Other critical reviewers included Andrew Hickey and Holly Matthies, who also suffer migraines. Dr. Damien Downing, president of the British Society for Ecological Medicine, provided me with information about migraines and various supplements. Dr. Abram Hoffer was gracious in responding to my e-mail questions. I am also grateful to Dr. Claus Hanke for his discussion of the role of orthomolecular medicine in normal medical practice. Dr. Gert Suitemaker and Elsedien de Groot from time to time provided helpful advice from their extensive knowledge of nutrition. Meleni Aldridge and Dr. Rob Verkerk continue to be supportive in promoting the role of nutrition in migraine and other aspects of health care.

This book would not exist without Andrew Saul, editor of *The Vitamin Cure* series, who was aware of my history of migraines and decided to aggravate the condition by suggesting I write about them. I accepted the challenge, as an opportunity to delve more closely into the underlying causes of migraine. For about three decades, I have been trying different remedies, some more effective than others, and writing this book allowed an intensified series of personal trials, along with the associated suffering and resultant findings.

INTRODUCTION

*If I wished to show a student the difficulties of
practice, I should give him a headache to treat.*
—OLIVER WENDELL HOLMES (1809–1894)

As anyone who suffers from migraines knows only too well, they
can occur at the most inconvenient times. A short time ago, I
was standing on a podium at a medical convention, before 300 or
so delegates, including world-renowned scientists and doctors. My
talk was controversial and certain members of the audience might
be eager to take advantage of any errors I might make. Normally, I
would relish such a challenge, but this time I had a migraine.

That morning, I had awakened around five o'clock, with a severe
pounding in the left side of my head. People don't normally sleep
through a migraine—some call it the "alarm clock headache," as the
pain is too intense to sleep. The veins in my head felt as though they
contained battery acid rather than blood, and my skull seemed to
expand and shrink with every heartbeat. Attempting to ease the
agony, I took a cocktail of drugs aimed at aborting the migraine, but
they had no effect. I then took a selection of painkillers to allow
myself just to function. The result was a slight dulling of the pain
and a substantial numbing of my faculties. For the next four hours,
I sat in a darkened room with my head wrapped in ice, with psychedelic colors and the high-pitched whine of tinnitus for company.

Although migraine pain is brutal, it was not my only problem.
Once in the conference room, I exhibited the first slide of my talk and

1

wondered whether I would find I was anomic. Anomia is the inability to remember nouns (the words used as names and labels). It is an atypical symptom of migraine, but happens to me often enough that I compensate for it in advance by putting essential words on the slides. My brain felt sluggish and the room seemed to darken, producing tunnel vision. Unfortunately, when the first slide appeared on the computer monitor, my vision was blurred—I could see two of everything and the text was unreadable. Turning my head to view the image projected for the audience, the glare from the screen increased my pain dramatically. However, at least I could read the words.

Looking into the darkened room, patches of color flooded my visual field, similar to effects reported for hallucinogenic drugs, and my ears continued to ring with high-pitched noise. From experience, I knew that I would need to avoid simple arithmetic calculations (paradoxically, complex logical and mathematical relations would be fine). Keep your sentences short and simple, I told myself. My left thumb started an involuntary twitch, so I had to use my right hand to change the slides. The urge to vomit had passed, but I felt dizzy and lightheaded. Apparently, I delivered my presentation in an acceptable manner, though, to be honest, I recall little about it.

Migraines can occur frequently and I have had many. My first, at the age of ten, was on a bus trip to Blackpool, a coastal resort in England. My mother told me I had travel sickness. For years, physicians told me my problems were caused by sinusitis. Eventually, I diagnosed my condition for myself. One of my reasons for writing this book was the opportunity to review medical progress on migraine and its treatment. In the process, I hoped I would find ways of reducing the number and severity of my own attacks. I am happy to report that I have managed to lower the intensity and frequency of my major headaches. Readers can have a reasonable expectation of similar benefit.

A MAJOR DISABILITY

Migraine is a major disability and one of the most incapacitating diseases. This book addresses the illness and provides an effective nutritional approach to treatment. Though painful, migraine and headache do not significantly increase the risk of death. Because of this, many people (medical professionals included) do not appreciate the seriousness of the condition.[1] Headache, and especially migraines, are major health problems, devastating people's lives and damaging the economy.

Almost half the population suffer from headaches. Migraine attacks interfere with employment, undermining the sufferer's career and financial prospects, as well as restricting family and social life. Migraineurs live in constant fear of the next attack.[2] Taking all causes of disease and disability into consideration, migraine is high on the list of conditions that take away useful years of a person's life. The World Health Organization (WHO) ranks headache as one of the ten most destructive conditions in terms of useful days lost.[3] Migraines specifically are ranked by the WHO as the nineteenth most devastating condition in terms of days lost to illness.[4] Since headaches are most common between the late teens and sixty years of age, there is a consequent loss to the economy and society[5]; about 25 million working or study days are lost to migraine each year in the United Kingdom alone.[6]

The pathologies of migraine and headache are difficult to study scientifically because of the complexity of investigating what is going on inside the brain and its surrounding tissues. However, recent research holds out the promise that developments in prevention and therapy may arise soon. Readers who are disabled by headaches can have reasonable expectations that their illness may be managed and they can get their lives back. This book aims to help people suffering from migraine headaches to reclaim time lost to this condition. While a cure for migraine is elusive, with appropriate nutritional support, sufferers' lives can be greatly improved.

THE LIMITS OF THE CONVENTIONAL APPROACH

Until recently, our understanding of migraines was misdirected. For centuries, it was considered a disease of the blood vessels. Later, doctors claimed it was related to levels of serotonin, the "happiness neurotransmitter" in the brain. More recently, migraine has been proposed to originate in the cortex of the brain, the brain stem, and the nerves that supply the face and head. Notwithstanding changes in understanding the underlying mechanisms, therapies based on earlier models have had some limited degree of success. For patients, however, the overall results have been discouraging.

Currently, a conventional migraine preventative drug considered to be excellent might give half the patients taking it an even chance of relief. That means about one quarter will gain reasonable benefit. Here, we define benefit as lowering the number of headaches by 50 percent. Neurologists claim that, given time, they have an strong chance of providing some level of relief to most of their patients. To achieve this, the patient will undergo a trial-and-error series of medications, each of which has a long list of potentially serious side effects. The aim is to see which drug, or combination of drugs, will provide noticeable benefit while minimizing unwelcome side effects. Conventional medicine provides little hope for a migraine sufferer who wants to avoid migraine attacks altogether. The widely prescribed paracetmol (acetaminophen), taken alone, will provide little if any relief.

Doctors might object to the last paragraph by arguing that modern drugs, such as the triptans, have revolutionized the process of aborting migraine attacks. There is some truth in this claim. However, simple nonsteroidal anti-inflammatory drugs (NSAIDs), such as aspirin, provide relief comparable to the much-hyped triptans at lower cost. When used correctly, combinations of NSAIDs, paracetamol, and caffeine can approach or even exceed the benefits of expensive triptan drugs. More importantly, changes in nutrition may provide even greater benefit.

THE PROMISE OF NUTRITIONAL TREATMENT

In terms of prevention, nutritional supplementation offers benefits that surpass the best that conventional medicine can provide. Particular supplements or nutrient combinations may be more effective than any drug offered by a physician, though we cannot know for sure because medical researchers have not conducted the necessary clinical trials. Where trial results of nutrients are available, they often equal current clinical medicine.

Nutrition should be the first line of defense for a migraine sufferer. This book describes nutritional approaches to both prevention and treatment, based on an orthomolecular perspective. Orthomolecular medicine involves the use of substances that are normally present in the body or are required for optimal functioning. Thus, practitioners use vitamins, minerals, and other associated nutritional supplements.

Since the orthomolecular approach may not be fully effective against migraine, this book also covers herbal remedies that may be helpful. These should be considered a second line of defense, to be used in addition to orthomolecular medicine for resistant migraines. In addition, there are some simple physical approaches, such as cooling the head, which also provide benefit without the side effects of drugs.

Where appropriate, the book includes a description of anti-migraine drugs. Sometimes the drug action illustrates what goes wrong in the body in migraine and is necessary to understand the disease. Drugs are appropriate as a last line of defense, for example, when a migraine attack breaks through. While a painkilling drug may be necessary to prevent or abort a migraine attack, nutrient supplementation can make this far less frequent. Some people on nutritional supplements and dietary change will achieve a complete cessation of migraines. Many will achieve fewer, less frequent, and less painful attacks.

Some supplements can terminate a migraine at an early stage; examples include large doses of niacin (a form of vitamin B_3) or curcumin, a derivative of turmeric. It is also possible to abort migraines using injections of magnesium sulfate, though this requires the help of a physician. Many physicians, even neurologists, are ignorant of this approach, so patients may find it difficult to obtain the support of a physician for these therapies. Hopefully, given time, the medical establishment will embrace the use of vitamins and other supplements for treating migraines and will develop a more scientific approach to the condition.

Migraine is difficult to treat effectively. There is no cure, though it is possible for sufferers to regain productive lives. This book suggests that nutrition should be the core treatment—dietary supplements can be as effective as the most powerful medicines, and result in fewer side effects.

CHAPTER 1

THE MIGRAINE EXPERIENCE

*That no one dies of a migraine seems to someone
deep in an attack an ambiguous blessing.*
—JOAN DIDION, AUTHOR OF *THE WHITE ALBUM*

Worldwide, more than 300 million people are afflicted by migraines; about one in six suffer at some time in their lives.[1] One in twenty lose at least a day a month and, for every 1,000 people in the population, three migraines occur each day.[2] The condition is more common in women, but men are also affected: migraine affects 15–18 percent of women and 6–8 percent of men.[3] However, the prevalence of migraines may be underestimated, as they are often misdiagnosed as sinusitis or some other condition.

Migraines usually begin at puberty and can extend throughout adult life. A study of 386 people over fourteen years of age found the lifetime prevalence to be 19.9 percent in males and 29.3 percent in females.[4] Although migraine can trouble young people and children, its occurrence peaks between the ages of thirty-five and forty-five years.

The higher prevalence in women appears to be a result of hormonal variations during the menstrual cycle. Over 12 million of the 20 million women in the United States with migraine have menstrual migraines.[5] In this type, women suffer migraines around the time of their period, although they can occur at other times of the month.[6] The cause is thought to be the drop in estrogen levels that happens during the period. Menstrual migraines may last longer, be more severe, and be harder to treat than regular migraines.[7]

The overall frequency of migraines in the affected population is reported as one or two a month; this is strongly influenced by the high proportion of menstrual migraines. For some, attacks are relatively mild and infrequent, but others experience them regularly. For the unlucky, migraines are a daily torture. This high frequency of attack is disabling, as migraines usually extend from several hours to several days.

There is a genetic component to migraines, so if a member of your family has the disease, you are at higher risk.[8] This suggests that migraine has probably been part of the human condition for a long time. Migraines have been known for several thousand years, which is as long as records exist. They have probably existed throughout human history and may account for trepanned holes found in Neolithic skulls. In 1660, William Harvey, the first Western doctor to describe the circulation of the blood, popularized trepanation (drilling holes in the skull) as a treatment for migraine.[9]

A Sumerian epic poem from 3000 B.C., which is believed to refer to migraine, reads: "The sick-eyed says not 'I am sick-eyed.' The sick-headed [says] not 'I am sick-headed'."[10] An early Egyptian remedy for migraine involved rubbing the aching side of the head with the head of a fish.[11] The Greek physician, Galen, the most influential doctor in the time of the Roman Empire and for centuries afterwards, described migraine as a painful affliction of one side of the head. He attributed it to a buildup of humors, or vapors, moving from the liver to the head.

MISUNDERSTOOD AND MISDIAGNOSED

In adults, symptoms include periodic attacks of disabling nauseous headache. These often occur with vomiting, along with intolerance to light and sound. The headaches are usually moderate, but can be severe. They are often one-sided, hence the name *migraine,* derived from the Greek word *hemicrania,* meaning "half the head." Migraine headaches pulsate, or throb, and are aggravated by physical activity.

Despite its long history, migraine is often misunderstood, misdiagnosed, and inadequately treated. Many sufferers do not seek medical help, being doubtful of doctors' ability to provide acceptable treatment. Far too many sufferers have experienced the skepticism of hostile doctors. People who have never suffered a migraine tend to think of it as a bad headache, so it can be frustrating to try to explain the difference. Women have described the pain as worse than childbirth; other people have said it is worse than a broken bone. Cluster headache, a form of migraine, is considered one of the most painful experiences possible.

Many people suffering migraine or headache do not receive effective health care.[12] In the United States and United Kingdom, only about half of patients with migraine had seen a doctor for the condition in the previous year.[13] Moreover, only two-thirds had been diagnosed accurately. These patients were often using over-the-counter medications, without prescription drugs. Despite this, two-thirds of respondents with migraine report searching for better treatment than their current drugs.[14]

Many sufferers are unaware that they have migraines. I was initially diagnosed, wrongly, as having chronic sinusitis. The sinuses are cavities in the frontal bones of the skull, which can become infected or inflamed. Since many atypical symptoms of migraine, such as frontal headache, eye pain or redness, and nasal congestion, also occur with sinus infection or inflammation, misdiagnosis is common. As many as 90 percent of headaches diagnosed as sinusitis may be migraines.[15] Partly, this confusion occurs because migraine involves the trigeminal nerves, which connect to the sinus region of the skull. The pain can thus appear to come from the sinus region, which responds to the affected nerve by becoming congested.

Because of the common misdiagnosis, many patients with "sinus headache" respond to triptan anti-migraine drugs rather than decongestants or antibiotics.[16] Anyone with chronic sinus or similar headaches should check the diagnosis—they may be suffering from migraine.

THE SYMPTOMS OF MIGRAINE

The symptoms of migraine vary with each individual. Some, for example, suffer flashing lights and other visual effects before an attack, while others may experience tinnitus (a high-pitched ringing in the ears). Migraines are often classified in terms of these early symptoms, though such categories may not reflect the severity of associated pain or disability.

The first problem facing a migraine sufferer is to get an accurate diagnosis. The main criterion for migraine is a headache with nausea. A person with a bad headache, who is also feeling sick or vomiting, most likely has a migraine. This chapter describes many of the features of migraines. Some sufferers may get few of these symptoms, other than the headache and nausea, while others will experience all of them, and perhaps even others that are not included in this limited description.

Prodrome

Many people report knowing that they are about to have a headache. About half of migraine sufferers describe a "prodrome" phase, which warns them of an impending attack. This occurs several hours, or even days, before a migraine. It includes symptoms of altered mood, depression, or euphoria.

Occasionally, subjects may know they will have a migraine tomorrow because they feel "dangerously great" today. For others, the prodrome is characterized by fatigue, excessive sleepiness, and yawning. The list of prodrome symptoms is long and variable and includes craving for specific foods (such as chocolate or ice cream), stiff neck muscles, changes in bowel movements, or increased urination. Over time, the patient may learn to recognize these symptoms and know that a migraine is on the way.

Aura

An aura is another warning signal than can precede a migraine, though generally by a period of minutes rather than the hours of the prodrome phase. Auras are highly variable and can take many forms. The classic aura involves zigzag hallucinations, often near the edge of the visual field. These geometric displays are sometimes quite dramatic: auras may appear like lightning bolts, sparks, flashes of light, or brilliant stars. Some people even lose their vision. An impending headache can also be signaled by a feeling of tingling or weakness on one or both side of the body. Some people have tinnitus. Occasionally, the person's speech or verbal ability is affected.

I experienced vivid "auras" for many years, during which time they occurred so frequently I thought everyone had them. In a darkened room, my visual field seemed covered in patches of bright colors, purple and orange clouds, that moved slowly about. I first noticed them when I was about ten years old, but paid them no heed.

Usually, an aura occurs before a headache, but they can also occur without a headache or can persist throughout an attack. An aura without a headache is described as an acephalgic or silent migraine. Such a condition is also known as ocular migraine, optical migraine, or even by the self-contradictory term *amigrainous migraine*. People with silent migraine may later develop standard migraine with headache.

Over the last century or so, people have used the term *aura* to describe the sensations and effects that precede migraines. However, for hundreds of years prior to this, aura was also applied to the feelings occurring before an epileptic seizure. This is interesting, as migraine and epilepsy have similar underlying mechanisms and the common use of the term brings out this link.

In addition to visual disturbances, there are many strange effects in the aura, such as changes in color perception, smell, or even feeling as though your hand is not part of your body (alien limb syndrome).[17] As related earlier, I suffer from a noticeable atypical symptom—I become anomic, meaning I find it hard to remember nouns. It is difficult to explain why your vocabulary has suddenly eluded you, and mildly embarrassing when you cannot remember a person's name. Consequently, I have developed a compensatory mechanism whereby I describe the nameless thing in terms of function. Often, I am able to maintain the flow without too many people realizing. However, one event was particularly awkward.

I had just completed a talk to several hundred scientists and physicians. The talk went well and, after leaving the stage, I was surrounded by professors and doctors who were asking me questions. There was no problem at first, since the questions concerned ideas that I had not covered in my presentation. Then came a dreaded question that I had no chance whatsoever of answering: someone asked me my name! I was dumbfounded, as I could not remember my own name. I was anomic and there was no way out. Saying I did not know who I was would have sounded crazy. I turned to another member of the group and added details concerning my response to a previous question. But the questioner persisted, "What is your name?" I racked my brain, but to no avail. I kept avoiding the question and talking to the others and must have appeared quite impolite. Luckily, a member of my university research team came forward and told the questioner my name.

Now, I no longer worry about such things. I can usually remember the term *anomia* or *atypical migraine* and simply explain that it is a minor neurological deficit. There are even reports of complete, temporary amnesia with migraine,[18] so just forgetting one's name is a relatively minor inconvenience.

A similar aura symptom I have experienced is variable dyslexia. Sometimes, I have no difficulty writing or spelling and am reasonably able to explain things. However, on other days, especially during my school years, I was apparently dyslexic. I found it hard to spell words and had difficulty constructing even a simple written sentence. What is more, it was impossible to tell before I started writing whether this was a dyslexic day or not. A second, presumably migraine-related experience that I have occurs with mathematics or computer science. Given a problem, I can sometimes see the answer right away, especially if it has some form of geometric representation. However, I cannot explain where the answer comes from. Moreover, only with the greatest difficulty can I derive or explain the result. This ability can occasionally be useful: in computing, for example, having a feel for the solution enables me to write code without the need for a preliminary design.

There have been many reports of people taking advantage of migraine effects. In some, a migraine aura may stimulate and enhance creative expression. The brilliant colors and line distortions in the paintings of Vincent van Gogh have been attributed to either migraine or temporolimbic epilepsy.[19] Temporolimbic epilepsy affects the deep structures (limbic system) and the side of the cortex (temporal lobe) in the brain. The cortex, a thin layer covering the outer surface of the two brain hemispheres, is believed to be the center for higher brain functions. The strange, somewhat psychedelic, swirling image in van Gogh's "Starry Night" painting might reflect how the painter saw the scene during a migraine aura. Similarly, Charles Lutwidge Dodgson's (Lewis Carroll) descriptions in his books *Alice's Adventures in Wonderland* and *Through the Looking-Glass* may be an interpretation of his view during a migraine aura or epileptic event. These related conditions may enhance perception of the surreal and the abstract.

Lists of famous artists, leaders, and scientists who have suffered from migraines include Miguel de Cervantes, Julius Caesar, Frédéric Chopin, Charles Darwin, Sigmund Freud, Ulysses S. Grant, Thomas Jefferson, Joan of Arc, Stephen King, Robert E. Lee, Karl Marx, Claude Monet, Friedrich Nietzche, Pablo Picasso, Edgar Allan Poe, and Pyotr Il'yich Tchaikovsky.[20] Although such a list could just reflect the frequency of the condition, it may offer a little consolation to artistically minded migraineurs.

How are auras generated? Doctors believe that an aura arises from a wave of electrical inhibition, which spreads across the cortex of the brain. At first, a wave of intense activity spreads through the nerve cells (neurons) in the cortex, including the areas that control vision. These active neurons need more energy, so blood flow is stimulated. Using magnetic resonance imaging (MRI), scientists have observed this increased blood flow in the brains of patients with migraine auras. Both migraine and epilepsy share this phenomenon of brain cell excitation. However, in migraine, the initial excitation leads to a depression of the nerve cells, whereas in epilepsy the excitation is synchronized over a large region of the brain.[21] In migraine, the excitatory phase is followed closely by inhibition of brain cell activity across the cortex. This depressed phase lasts a comparatively long time, during which the brain cells are relatively unexcitable. As the inhibited neurons are inactive, they require less oxygen, so local blood flow may be reduced.

Importantly, nerve cell excitability in migraine is particularly associated with a single chemical neurotransmitter called glutamate.[22] Glutamate is the primary excitatory neurotransmitter that brain cells use to communicate with each other; it causes brain cells to become more active. Glutamate functions by attaching to the NMDA (N-methyl D-aspartate) receptors. (The name refers to another chemical, aspartate, which also binds to these receptors.) NMDA receptors control channels into nerve cells, which affect nerve cell excitability.

This description might seem unnecessarily technical, but it is relevant because glutamate, aspartate, and similar migraine-inducing chemicals are widely available in the modern diet.

The Attack

A migraine attack can be a severe and debilitating experience. As Joan Didion wrote, "The actual headache, when it comes, brings with it chills, sweating, nausea, a debility that seems to stretch the very limits of endurance. That no one dies of migraine seems, to someone deep into an attack, an ambiguous blessing."[23] Unfortunately, people who have not experienced migraine often fail to understand the discomfort of the sufferer, thinking it is "only a headache." This incapacity to appreciate the problem continues to drive some modern research.

The sufferer may be rendered helpless, confined to a darkened room and unable to move. Despite this, the severity of the symptoms is often underestimated, even by experienced researchers. Since the brain is enclosed within the skull, finding out exactly what is happening during a migraine is, as we shall see, a challenging scientific endeavor. Throughout a migraine attack, the brain's blood flow, use of energy, and electrical activity are all markedly altered; the brain, and often the whole body, can suffer inflammation. As we follow the migraine story, these profound, extensive, though strangely benign, changes in the brain will be made clear. Migraine is a neurological condition but, like many conditions that are common in women, migraines have often been dismissed as a psychological condition. Migraineurs are often thought to be overstating their "headache," as if the pain were an illusion.

A recent theory by leading researcher Peter Goadsby is that the pain of migraine is an illusion created within the brain.[24] According to him, the migraine brain is more sensitive to incoming stimuli—

light, sound, and smell are all more intense—and this explains the aura that some patients experience before an attack. The signals coming into the brain overload the system, overflowing into other channels. This signal overflow affects areas of the brain that process pain and other sensory perceptions. The result, according to Goadsby, is an acute brain overload, with an "illusion" of pain that we call migraine. As we present further information concerning what happens during a migraine attack, it will become clear that, although this "migraine as an illusion" theory is interesting, it does not fit the available evidence.

In support of Goadsby's idea, migraineurs are generally more sensitive to pain and process sensory information a little differently from other people. A normal person responds to a repetitive sound or image by habituating to the signal: as data is repeated, it is ignored. However, in the migraineur's brain, repeated signals are not damped down in this way. The resultant signal overload in migraine is, in some ways, related to a theory about hallucinogenic drugs such as LSD. Such drugs have been claimed to reduce the inhibition of sensory signals into the brain, resulting in a "psychedelic experience." Some aspects of migraine are similar, in that there are distortions of visual, auditory, taste, smell, and other signals from the body, which could also be caused by signal overload.

The internal information-processing mechanism is only part of the process. Focusing on perception may give the impression that a migraine is not a real disease but rather an illusion. However, there is no evidence to suggest that migraine pain is psychological. Even if migraines are a disorder of the brain, they have substantial peripheral effects. Bleeding gums, red eyes, blocked nose, and joint pain and inflammation are signs that migraine affects the whole system.

Many migraineurs will resent the implication that the illness is illusory. This theory takes us back to the medical problem, where doctors, often unable to provide effective help, dismiss the disease. Once again, Joan Didion puts it well: "I had no brain tumor, no eyestrain, no high blood pressure, nothing wrong with me at all: I simply had migraine headaches, and migraine headaches were, as everyone who did not have them knew, imaginary."[25]

The idea that the pain of a migraine is "not really happening" is just plain silly. The suggestion that the brain generates an "illusion" of pain, even if it were correct, would not mean that the pain experience is not real. All pain is experienced within the brain. Break a bone in your leg and pain fibers will carry a signal to the brain. The brain will interpret the signal as pain, but the experience is generated centrally. Ironically, it may be easier to modify the experience of pain from a broken leg than that of a migraine.

To put the level of migraine pain into perspective, consider the results of a Gallup Organization poll of 1,007 migraineurs conducted for Cerenex Pharmaceuticals.[26] The pain of an attack was sufficiently intense that 35 percent of sufferers indicated that they had wished they were dead. Migraine was rated more painful than childbirth (19 percent), a broken bone (28 percent), arthritis (33 percent), athletic injuries (42 percent), and a bad burn (42 percent). It was also reported that one in three people missing work through migraine did not mention the true cause, as it would be considered just a headache. This popular view is unfortunate because in a migraine, the brain is malfunctioning and there are deleterious effects throughout the body.

Postdrome

On the day following a migraine, the person often feels depressed, "beaten up" or washed out, and has no appetite. The sufferer may need time to recover. The drained and listless response during this postdrome phase may interfere with normal activities. The sufferer has no energy and little internal drive. Some people report that they occasionally feel euphoric or refreshed following an attack. In others, headache and other symptoms may persist at a low level.

THE GENETICS OF MIGRAINE

Migraine is in part hereditary. As is usual with poorly understood medical conditions, the cause is generally described as multifactorial. Such explanations are typically unhelpful. Medical conditions, behavior patterns, or related events in which the cause is unknown are often considered to have a large number of related risk factors.

The term *multifactorial* frequently reflects a lack of knowledge and, in many cases, the supposed risk factors may be chance associations.

A large number of factors are loosely associated with migraine. Identical twins are more likely to both suffer migraines than are non-identical twins, for example. However, the disease is not associated with a single gene. A number of influences may alter the genetic predisposition. The disease is not purely genetic, since one identical twin can have the disease, while the other does not.

A relatively rare form of the illness, familial hemiplegic migraine, sheds light on the underlying genetics. This form runs in families and is associated with one-sided paralysis. In these people, certain genes are mutated; these code for calcium channels, which help control brain cells by maintaining their electrical state.[27] The channels involved in hemiplegic migraine are normally closed, but are opened (activated) when the electrical difference (voltage) between the cell and its exterior drops. The familial hemiplegic migraine mutation may make the sufferer more sensitive to environmental factors.[28]

Migraine genetics are complex. Families suffering from migraine may possess different genetic influences based on the involvement of several genes. However, as we have seen, the genetics do suggest the involvement of calcium channels. In particular, the NMDA channel provides a key to the nutritional control of migraine.

Migraine may be a side effect of human evolution, a problem that has not had time to be eliminated from the gene pool. It is also possible that migraine (and other widespread diseases, such as schizophrenia) have provided evolutionary benefit at some time in the past.[29] Migraineurs can be rendered almost helpless during an attack, which would have subjected them to enormous biological selection pressures. If sufferers were not to be wiped out, any advantage would need to be large enough to overcome the disadvantages of migraines and it would need to be subtle, otherwise it would be obvious.

One suggestion is that migraine brains are particularly sensitive, and the symptoms of migraine may force sufferers to withdraw from potentially harmful situations. Charles Darwin himself suffered from migraines; the enforced periods of silence and solitude during migraine attacks may have allowed him the time and space to develop his theories of evolution.

Another possible evolutionary advantage relates to the finding that migraineurs are exquisitely responsive to a variety of environmental stimuli. This may lead them to give increased attention to sensory stimuli such as light, noise, and smell. As a result, they might be more likely to notice environmental threats and would tend to avoid dangerous situations.

CHAPTER 2

A SEARCH FOR CAUSES

*I am sick of diseases, I want to know origins
and processes. . . . If we are to prevent disease
it is to the beginning of the chain of
accumulating stresses that we must look.*
—SIR THOMAS CLIFFORD ALLBUTT (1836–1925)

THE MIGRAINE BRAIN

While the brain itself does not feel pain, the large trigeminal nerve is sensitive. This nerve is responsible for sensation in the face and for certain motor functions, such as chewing and swallowing. It transmits pain signals from the meningeal membranes that surround the brain. Pain from the meninges, or the associated blood vessels, is transmitted to the brain stem. In the aura phase, a wave of spreading depression in the brain's cortex leads to inflammation, which overstimulates the trigeminal nerve. This results in the release of glutamate and nitric oxide (NO), which may cause the trigeminal nerve to transmit pain signals. NO is a local hormone or chemical messenger; it is essential to the proper health and functioning of our bodies.

Signals from the trigeminal nerve are modified by the brain stem. The wave of spreading depression during a migraine aura may be secondary to overloading the brain stem with signals. Three small areas in the brain stem (called the raphe nucleus, the locus coeruleus, and the periaqueductal gray) are excited during migraine attacks. These centers are involved in modulating pain, emotional responses, and alertness; in particular, they inhibit signals from the trigeminal nerve. If these nuclei fail to damp down such signals, they may be transmitted to the brain as pain.

The activity of these brain stem centers, especially the raphe nucleus, depends critically on the ion channels in their nerve cells. The raphe nucleus releases serotonin and noradrenaline. Since serotonin was considered the happiness chemical, drug companies targeted it for the creation of antidepressants. Over time, it became apparent that Prozac and other SSRI (selective serotonin reuptake inhibitor) antidepressants were largely ineffective.[1] The role of serotonin in depression has been overemphasized, as it has with migraine.

In evolutionary terms, the brain stem is an old structure, as much an extension of the spinal cord as part of the brain. The main motor and sensory innervations to the face and neck, via the cranial nerves, arise from the brain stem. Motor (movement) and sensory signals to and from the rest of the body—including motor control, touch, vibration, pain, temperature, and the senses of movement and position—travel through the brain stem. Sensory, pain, and inflammation signals from the head arrive at the brain stem via the trigeminal nerve. The brain stem regulates brain function, sleep, and helps maintain consciousness. The wide and varied bodily symptoms that can be associated with migraine may result from the involvement of the brain stem, with its many diverse functions.

Brain imaging has shown that regions of the brain stem are active during migraine attacks[2] and cluster headaches. Migraine triggers often induce excitation in the nerve cells of the cortex and brain stem; this may prevent the brain stem from blocking excess sensory information.[3] Nerves then convey signals back to the brain areas that may have originally triggered the brain stem. This feedback can drive the migraine attack for hours or even days.[4]

ADVANCES IN MIGRAINE DIAGNOSIS

Migraines are subtle and do not appear to be associated with major brain damage. In some ways, migraine is harder to investigate than life-threatening conditions, such as cancer or heart disease. Animal experiments are also of limited value: a rat cannot tell you if it is having a migraine or give an account of the symptoms. Fortunately, there are ways to gain insight into what happens when a person has a migraine. Doctors perform clinical examinations and take samples of blood or spinal fluids, which can be examined chemically. They study the pharmacology of drugs that prevent or abort migraine, many of which have known mechanisms that suggest the underlying pathology. Scientists also research the substances that act as migraine triggers. They use electroencephalography (EEG) to record brain electrical activity from the patient's scalp. However, these indirect methods of investigation are limited, as they do not give direct insight into the disease. Consequently, the cause of the illness is still not fully established, despite migraines being both common and debilitating.

Recently, magnetic resonance imaging (MRI) has enabled doctors to visualize the brain relatively safely. One particular form, functional MRI, allows the doctor to view changes in brain's blood flow as they happen. In active parts of the brain, blood flow increases when the person is thinking or responding to a stimulus. By measuring the blood flow, the more active parts of the brain can be identified. Researchers have noticed that increased blood flow in a region of the brain is associated with it becoming more electrically active. These observations produce a chicken and egg conundrum: it is often not clear whether the blood is flowing faster because of the increased electrical activity, or because the increase in blood flow alters the behavior of the brain cells. Interestingly, the observed increase in blood flow is far greater than needed to provide additional energy for processing.[5] The blood nourishes the brain cells but may also be intimately involved in information processing. Notably, changes in the brain's blood flow are characteristic of migraines.

The introduction of functional MRI has shown that some established ideas about what goes wrong during a migraine were mistaken.[6] As a result, we now have more reasonable models for the disease process. However, before we look at current ideas of the brain in migraine, we will explain how some older ideas have been superseded.

CONVENTIONAL MODELS OF MIGRAINE

Blood Vessel Theory

The blood vessel theory of migraine replaced that of the eminent Greek physician, Galen (129–200 A.D.), who followed Hippocrates in attributing the condition to vapors in the head. Hippocrates (circa 460–370 B.C.) thought that "humors," fluids or vapors circulating in the body, rose from the liver to the head causing migraine. These ideas were central to Western medicine for the next thousand years, and his migraine theory lasted until the seventeenth century.

In about the year 1150, Hildegard of Bergen suggested: "Migraine stems from the black bile and from all the other bad humors that are in a person. It strikes in the middle of the head and not the entire head, so that sometimes it is located on the right side and sometimes on the left. . . . Migraine has such a force within itself that, if it occupied the entire head all at once, a person could not withstand it."[7]

Later, the English physician William Harvey (1578–1657) described the circulation of the blood. He was not the first—a thirteenth-century Persian physician, Ibn al-Nafis, had described it earlier—but this was not known in the West. Harvey's model of blood flow was used to develop ideas concerning migraine headaches. Thomas Willis (1621–1675), another English doctor, is famous for the ring of large blood vessels in the brain that carries his name, the circle of Willis. He proposed that migraine arises from a swelling of blood vessels in the head. This idea was the start of the vascular theory of migraine. For centuries, migraines were thought to be a disorder of blood vessels in the brain and head. The brain has a massive requirement for oxygen and nutrients, delivered by its blood vessels. Despite weighing little over a kilogram, when a person is at rest, the brain consumes about a fifth of the body's oxygen and energy.[8]

For many years, the idea that migraines originated in the arteries and veins seemed reasonable, considering the size and number of such vessels in the brain. The vascular theory remained the leading explanation until at least the 1980s. This model suggested that migraine pain stems from stress in the blood vessels in, or near, the brain. New York physician Harold Wolff (1898–1962) was a recent advocate of the idea.[9] Since the brain itself does not contain pain receptors, the idea that migraine pain originates in or around the blood vessels, which do have pain receptors, made sense.

According to the blood vessel theory, the pain in migraine arises directly from dilation and stretching of blood vessels in the brain. These blood vessels are thought to be hyper-excitable, responding abnormally to signals. Initially, the blood vessels were thought to contract in a spasm, reducing blood flow to the brain. Reduction in blood flow to the visual areas was believe to cause the aura and associated visual effects.[10] When a blood vessel tires after contracting, or otherwise relaxes, it dilates. In one version of the theory, expansion of the vessel following the contraction stretches its pain receptors, giving rise to the headache. Each beat of the heart then increases the pressure in the blood vessel, generating a throbbing pain. In another version, expansion creates gaps between the cells of the blood vessel wall, allowing fluid and chemicals to pass and breaching the blood-brain barrier. The chemicals leach into the surrounding tissue, causing local inflammation and pain.

The blood vessels in question are in and around the meninges, the three layers of membranes that enclose the brain. One reason this model was taken so seriously was the clinical similarity of migraine to the well-known infectious disease, meningitis (inflammation of the meninges). In migraine, the meninges may be inflamed, causing the blood vessels to expand, though there is no infection.[11] The symptoms of both migraine and meningitis include painful headache, sensitivity to light, stiff neck, and vomiting. Unlike meningitis, however, migraine is relatively benign and causes little apparent long-term damage.

The blood vessel theory seems reasonable but it is contradicted by recent findings. Fluid flow through a tube, such as a blood vessel, is highly sensitive to changes in diameter. Even slight blood vessel constriction would greatly lower the flow of blood and oxygen to the corresponding areas of the brain. However, recent MRI brain scans show that the blood vessels expand before a migraine, and correspondingly, the blood flow increases rather than decreases. The increase in blood flow can be large, perhaps three times the normal resting values. During the actual headache, the blood flow returns to normal or even below normal.

The blood vessel theory continued until the discovery of this inconsistent evidence in the last twenty years. One reason for its popularity was it explained many of the symptoms of migraine, and drugs that acted on blood vessels were partially effective treatments. Despite being incorrect, the blood vessel theory generated apparently beneficial therapies. Thus, many anti-migraine drugs are targeted on the blood vessels in the brain: some make the blood vessels less responsive to stress; others, such as ergotamine, constrict the blood vessels.[12]

Ergotamine takes its name from ergot, a dark-purple fungal spike that is found on rye and closely related plants. The drug, which is derived from ergot, has the power to constrict blood vessels. There may be another explanation for its anti-migraine effect: ergotamine is related to LSD-25, a powerful hallucinogen, and acts on the brain's serotonin receptors. Because of this action, scientists interested in migraine switched their attention to drugs that affect the brain's use of serotonin; we will examine this idea in more detail in the next section.

A different approach to the blood vessel theory involved using drugs to make the blood vessels less responsive to stress. Doctors thought that stopping the initial constriction of blood vessels might prevent a migraine. Typically, beta-blocker drugs, such as propranolol, are used to prevent high blood pressure. The beta-blockers act on blood vessels and lower the heart rate and blood pressure. By making blood vessels in the head less responsive to stress, beta-blockers were believed to lower the incidence of migraines, or reduce their intensity, in some patients.[13] However, although they are occasionally effective in preventing migraines, beta-blockers may work by acting directly on the brain rather than via the blood vessels.[14]

During a migraine, blood flow may increase in the cerebral hemispheres and brain stem.[15] However, recent brain imaging studies indicate that this dilation of the blood vessels occurs because of the migraine rather than as a cause. Indeed, blood vessel dilation may be a side issue.[16] Magnetic resonance imaging suggests that changes in blood flow seen in migraine attacks and cluster headaches are a response to pain and do not cause the condition.[17]

The vascular explanation of migraine is no longer considered valid. The changes in the diameter of blood vessels appear to be a consequence of events happening within the brain, not their cause. Despite this, the blood vessel theory is still accepted by many doctors, as the drugs targeted on blood vessels are partially effective and it takes time for new ideas to become established. We need to look elsewhere to understand what happens to the brain in migraine.

Serotonin Theory

After the failure of the blood vessel explanation, scientists suggested that low levels of serotonin, a neurotransmitter sometimes described as "the happiness molecule," might cause migraines.[18] Serotonin and other neurotransmitters are involved in signaling between brain cells. Transmitters and their receptors are affected by various drugs and were therefore the target for many theories of brain disorders and treatments. This led to decades of research attempting to relate neurotransmitters to brain function and disease. The serotonin theory of migraine began in the 1950s and tailed off in the 1990s.

In migraine, the serotonin theory is supported by the observation that blocking the synthesis of 5-hydroxytryptophan (5-HTP), a precursor of serotonin, could produce migraine symptoms. The alternative name for serotonin, 5-hydroxytriptamine (5-HT), indicates the similarity between these two molecules. However, while a shortage of serotonin can produce migraines, so can many other stresses, such as caffeine withdrawal. Moreover, administration of 5-HTP as a nutritional supplement that increases brain serotonin is beneficial but has limited effectiveness in migraine prevention and does not appear to abort migraine attacks.

Triptan drugs, such as sumatriptan, which are effective in aborting migraines, act on a serotonin receptor called 5-HT1. There are several types of receptors for serotonin in the brain, and drugs are targeted to act on specific receptors. However, these drugs also have other effects that can explain their action, as will be described later. In short, the serotonin explanation for migraines emerges from the neurotransmitter model but does not have convincing or specific supporting evidence.

Inflammation Theory

Migraine is now thought to be a result of inflammation.[19] Preventing the inflammation can prevent or abort a migraine.[20] Indeed, most diseases involve inflammation, oxidation, and free radical damage, and migraine is no exception.[21] The pain in migraine may arise directly from inflammation of nerves.[22] However, the nerves themselves may be the source of inflammation. Inflammatory chemicals are released near sensory nerve fibers, which activate pain receptors in the covering of the brain. The inflammation causes local blood vessels to dilate, by releasing nitric oxide, for example. This explanation illustrates how findings related to the blood vessel theory of migraine have been incorporated into more modern approaches.

With migraines, we are focused on a nerve in the head called the trigeminal nerve. Female hormones, such as estrogen, can sensitize the trigeminal nerve to inflammation.[23] The trigeminal nerve is one of twelve cranial nerves that mostly serve the head and neck, and enter the brain stem at the base of the brain. It is the main carrier of migraine pain signals, and stimulation of the trigeminal nerve can also produce local inflammation. Conventional anti-migraine drugs such as the aspirin-like NSAIDs, triptans,[24] and ergot derivatives[25] can block this inflammation and bring about relief from an attack. Later, we will describe how some supplements can provide an anti-inflammatory action equal to or greater than the NSAIDs.

Triptan drugs, such as sumatriptan, were developed with the aim of blocking serotonin receptors but may actually work by preventing inflammation. Drugs can have more than one action in the body and this is particularly true of anti-migraine medications, which were often developed for other conditions. One small protein involved in migraine inflammation, called calcitonin gene-related peptide (CGRP), is of particular interest.[26] Calcitonin is a hormone involved in regulating calcium in the blood. CGRP is associated with calcitonin but is involved with both inflammation and pain, and it is now a major target for development of new anti-migraine drugs.

In migraines, inflammation dilates blood vessels, mediated by the CGRP hormone. CGRP is one of the most powerful dilators of blood vessels known to occur naturally in the body. When nerve stimulation produces inflammation, CGRP is released, expanding the small blood vessels and making them leaky.[27] This hormone thus links the inflammatory model of migraine to the earlier blood vessel theory.

CGRP can cause migraine. During migraine attacks, CGRP increases in venous blood coming from the brain.[28] Originally, researchers did not know whether CGRP caused the migraines or was a side issue being produced by the attack. They therefore compared the effect of injecting CGRP to that of a placebo in ten migraine patients. Within an hour of the CGRP injection, the experimental group had a higher headache score than the controls, a highly significant result. Within twelve hours of the injection, all the CGRP patients suffered headaches, compared with only one of the placebo group. Once again, the result was highly significant. Three of the patients receiving CGRP were classified as having migraine without aura, but no placebo patient was classified as having a migraine. They concluded that CGRP may play a causative role in spontaneous headache and migraines.

The anti-migraine effects of triptan drugs may be a lucky side effect. In addition to dilating blood vessels, CGRP affects several inflammatory processes.[29] When sumatriptan is given to abort a migraine, in addition to blocking the action of serotonin it also lowers levels of CGRP.[30] Triptan drugs inhibit release of CGRP and this reduction is proportional to the headache relief.[31] In a migraine attack, the release of both glutamate and CGRP, causing inflammation of the trigeminal nerve, is controlled by calcium channels and influenced by serotonin signaling.[32] If it is eventually confirmed that these "breakthrough" drugs work indirectly as anti-inflammatory agents, it will be clear that they were developed for what later proved to be an unwanted side effect.

Findings such as these illustrate the ignorance associated with modern drug development. Effective agents can be produced through research and development, despite a misunderstanding of the underlying mechanisms. Drugs that abort migraines by interfering with CGRP release in the trigeminal nerve, without the side effects of serotonin blockage, are the new horizon for anti-migraine therapy.[33]

Since CGRP may be an essential component of migraines, inhibition of this molecule may abort an attack. Indeed, drugs that antagonize the action of CGRP can abort a migraine attack.[34] In one study of acute migraine attacks, the overall response to a CGRP inhibitor was 66 percent compared with 27 percent for the placebo. The response was rapid, with a difference between the drug and the placebo at thirty minutes, increasing through the four-hour period following administration.[35]

Brain Energy Theory

Migraine reflects a problem with the energy supply to the brain. In the days leading up to and following an attack, migraine sufferers often feel lethargic and drained; this may be a sign of a decreased cellular energy supply. Brain cells that lack sufficient energy may be unable to respond to normal stresses or stimuli, leading to hypersensitivity and migraines. When cellular energy is decreased, the toxic effects of excitotoxins (poisons that stimulate brain cells to death) and free radicals increase dramatically.[36]

We need to breathe continuously to supply the brain with oxygen. Other organs need oxygen but the brain's need is dramatic: lack of oxygen for just a few minutes will result in brain death. Brain cells are dependent on a continuous supply of oxygen and nutrients to provide energy. By contrast, muscle and fat cells can exist far longer than brain cells without oxygen for metabolism. Lack of energy makes brain cells more sensitive to stress induced by trigger factors.[37] In addition, the protective supply of antioxidants, essential for cells to withstand stress, needs energy and would be impaired.

The brain's energy supply depends on mitochondria, which are tiny structures within the cells. Mitochondria are rather similar in shape and size to bacteria but occur normally within the large cells of animals and plants. Early in evolution, it is believed, cells were infected with bacteria-like organisms; these perhaps acted as parasites but eventually entered into a fully symbiotic (mutually beneficial) relationship with the host cell. The host cell protected the bacteria from a hostile environment, while the bacteria provided an efficient energy supply. Because they are now part of the animal cell, children inherit their mitochondria from their mothers. In view of this, it is interesting to note that there is a slight maternal bias in the heritability of migraine.[38]

Mitochondrial damage may be genetic in origin or could be a result of poisoning. Notably, some drugs are a major cause of mitochondrial damage: psychotropic drugs can damage mitochondria, as can paracetamol. One line of response to mitochondrial damage is the use of targeted nutrient therapy. Antioxidants, such as coenzyme Q_{10}, alpha-lipoic acid, or N-acetyl-cysteine (NAC), hold promise for improving mitochondrial functioning. However, there are large gaps in our knowledge. A rational approach is to understand the mechanisms underlying mitochondrial damage in specific medications and then attempt to counteract their deleterious effects with nutritional therapies.

Some mitochondrial diseases cause migraine symptoms. Migraine is a feature of MELAS syndrome, which stands for mitochondrial myopathy, encephalopathy, lactic acidosis, and stroke-like episodes. MELAS is a progressive degenerative disease of the nervous system, which involves migraine-like headaches and vomiting. Strokes, which often occur toward the back of the brain, are a primary symptom of MELAS, though fortunately they are only a rare complication of migraines. The white matter abnormalities seen in brain scans of migraine patients could be a result of mitochondrial problems.[39]

Similar headaches on one side of the head are reported in another mitochondrial disease, called MERRF, myoclonic epilepsy with ragged-red fibers.[40] MERRF sufferers exhibit short stature and progressive, jerky epileptic seizures. When their cells are viewed under the microscope, the mitochondria in muscle fibers are seen to clump together, giving the appearance of "ragged-red fibers." The mitochondrial defects in this disease are thought to be associated with genetic damage.[41]

Migraines may involve problems with the mitochondrial energy supply. There can be depression of enzymes associated with mitochondria in muscles and platelets.[42] Magnetic resonance studies have shown a defective energy metabolism in the brain and muscle of migraineurs.[43] Migraine reflects an underlying deficit, involving lack of energy, sensitivity to excitotoxins, oxidation, and inflammation. Fortunately, this metabolic deficit may be addressed with nutritional supplementation.

MIGRAINE BRAINS ARE DIFFERENT

None of the conventional models for the cause of migraine provides a complete explanation. However, they might be parts of a larger system. Migraine may well be caused by a positive feedback loop: linking different mechanisms, enhancing the signals, and ultimately resulting in pain and other symptoms. Viewing migraine in this way enables a more holistic approach to its treatment, and we can see that vitamins and other supplements provide a more rational approach to migraine therapy.

Migraine brains are unusual. People with migraine appear to have an increased thickness of cortex in areas of their brains that are associated with processing movement.[44] However, researchers found no difference between sufferers with or without aura. One of these movement areas had previously been found to be the source of spreading depression in a person who had migraine with aura. The study also found differences in the area's associated white matter. Brain tissues are usually described in terms of gray and white matter. The bundles of nerve fibers that transfer information between different regions of the brain appear white, relative to the gray matter of the cortex and other highly cellular areas.

Another study indicated that migraineurs have a thicker somatosensory cortex,[45] an area of the brain that processes incoming signals from the skin, muscles, and bones. The greatest increase in thickness was in the area where signals from the head and face are processed. This area of maximal increase responds to signals from the trigeminal nerve and processes signals related to migraine.

Increased cortical thickness may be a result of repeated migraine attacks. The brain increases in thickness in response to use and thins in degenerative diseases, such as Alzheimer's disease. This is the source of the oft-stated "use it or lose it" advice for maintaining or building brain function.[46] Overstimulation of these signal-overloaded areas in the cortex could produce a corresponding increase in the tissue size. Alternatively, people with migraine may be particularly sensitive to normal brain signals because they have an over-developed cortex. Such sensitivity could explain the pain reported from the joints, skin, and other areas of the body during a migraine attack.

Migraine brains respond to sensory input with overload, inflammation, and pain. The brain's internal control mechanisms break down. There are many triggers for migraine but one of the more interesting is that images, paintings, patterns, and light effects can cause headaches. Some images, for example, of radiating lines with a repeating pattern can trigger a migraine attack or photosensitive epilepsy.[47] Images that generate discomfort appear to have a number of high-contrast repeating lines that are close together[48]; simple striped patterns can induce headaches. In some ways, the disturbing pictures are similar to the visual experience in migraine with aura. Indeed, some artists, such as Debbie Ayles, who paint images inspired by their migraines, can find people complaining that the images are uncomfortable to view and give them headaches.[49] The underlying reasons why viewing aura-like images produces migraines is unclear. However, the images may stimulate the visual cortex of the brain in a similar way to the initial stages of a migraine. That it goes on to generate a full migraine shows how a simple signal can break down the brain's internal controls.

Historically, models used to explain the migraine process have been limited by the difficulty in investigating what goes on in the sick tissues. As we shall see, these models for the disease can be combined in a single explanation that shows how vitamins and other dietary change provide the rational approach to therapy.

BREAKDOWN IN THE CONTROL SYSTEMS

Migraines may be due to a problem with the brain's internal controls. Rather than there being one unique cause, migraine may be a common response to any number of breakdowns in signal, pain, or inflammation controls. Control systems are central to understanding biological disease mechanisms, but they have tended to be overlooked by modern medicine.[50] The current medical paradigm promotes the statistical and genetic explanations of social medicine.[51] The science of control, known as cybernetics, is as robust an explanation as the most rigorous forms of evidence-based medicine. Notably, individual control is central to the philosophy of orthomolecular medicine and the use of vitamins and other nutrients in treating disease.

Normally, our bodies keep themselves running within tight limits by means of a biological mechanism called homeostasis. This is analogous to the mechanism of a thermostat used to control a central heating system. If the temperature of the room falls below a set level, the thermostat turns the heating on. When the radiators have raised the temperature above the thermostat setting, it switches the heating off. In systems theory, this process is called negative feedback, because the thermostat causes a change in the opposite direction to what it has detected (e.g., increased temperature leads to turning off the radiators, which reduces the temperature).

Similarly, homeostasis helps our bodies keep our internal temperature relatively constant and controls many other systems, such as blood pressure, fluid intake, or blood sugar levels. Homeostasis depends on negative feedback, which is a powerful and useful means of maintaining equilibrium. In negative feedback, the output is fed back into the system, smoothing out fluctuations as deviations and perturbations are damped down. Many of the systems in our bodies, such as heart rate, depend on negative feedback to keep us alive.

In the example above, increasing the temperature caused the thermostat to turn the radiators off, whereas decreasing it caused them to be switched on. But suppose the opposite were to happen: the radiators were turned up when the temperature increased. The house would soon overheat and eventually the boiler might blow up! This is an example of positive feedback, which can easily become catastrophically unstable.

Positive feedback occurs when a system responds to change by altering in the same direction, amplifying the perturbation. Rather than being a generally useful process, positive feedback gives an explosive response. Indeed, both chemical and nuclear explosions depend on positive feedback amplification. While the normal brain depends on negative feedback to maintain its healthy state, a migraine attack corresponds to a state of explosive positive feedback.

EXPLOSIVE FEEDBACK

Explosive positive feedback causes a migraine attack. An information loop connects the brain stem to the cortex and back again by way of the trigeminal nerve. Signals travel around the head and brain, being amplified to generate pain. If we start with a signal from the brain stem, it stimulates the NMDA (N-methyl D-aspartate) and other receptors in the brain's cortex. The cortical brain cells respond with fleeting excitation followed by cortical spreading depression, which leads to inflammation in the blood vessels and tissues. This amplified signal is then picked up by the trigeminal nerve, which becomes inflamed and reports pain in the scalp, head, and face. The trigeminal nerve similarly amplifies the signal and returns it to the brain stem to start the cycle once more.

A disturbance in any part of this system can initiate positive feedback, which magnifies the effect and ultimately generates a migraine attack. Almost any stimulus can send the system into a debilitating headache. According to this view, migraines happen because of a failure to prevent the positive feedback. The existence of positive feedback suggests that once a migraine is initiated, it may grow in intensity, rapidly becoming more severe. A positive feedback loop can accelerate the process, expanding a small signal to one that overloads the system. Once the headache starts it will be difficult to stop. Most people do not suffer migraines because they have damping mechanisms that prevent the amplification of pain and other signals. Migraine sufferers are highly susceptible to sensory overload because the damping mechanisms in their brain stems are less effective.

The bodily symptoms of migraine can be understood as a failure in finely balanced internal controls in the brain and nervous system. The central nervous system forms a major control system for the body; when a migraine occurs, its internal controls go awry, triggering responses throughout the body. Signals from any source may be magnified. Muscles, bones, and joints may ache, leaving a normally healthy young person feeling old and arthritic.

One common symptom of migraine is that the person's stomach shuts down in a defensive response. Sickness and nausea can be caused by poisoning, so preventing absorption from the gut is an evolutionary adaptation in times of stress and sickness. Unfortunately, for the migraineur, this may mean that painkillers taken to ease a headache may not be absorbed while the attack is in progress. After the attack, the tablets may be absorbed all at once, with obvious dangers considering the toxicity of some anti-migraine drugs. In this case, the evolutionary adaptation prevents benefit from medication, which is not absorbed until the symptoms subside, but amplifies the drugs' toxicity and side effects.

If we consider migraine as a positive feedback loop, many apparently conflicting data on its pathology and triggers can be reconciled. The migraine feedback loop is overloaded by neural signals, local free radicals, pain, stress, or inflammation. It does not matter if the initial stimulus is a disturbance in the cortex, inflammation in the trigeminal nerve, or failure to damp a sensory input in the brain stem. The signal enters the feedback pathway and is explosively enhanced with every cycle of the system.

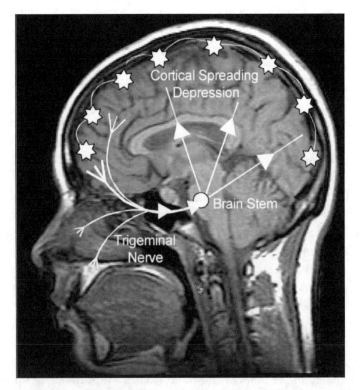

The explosive feedback signal in migraine spreads from the brain stem to the surface of the brain (cortical spreading depression) and back to the brain stem via the trigeminal nerve.

MIGRAINE TRIGGERS

According to the systems model, the varied triggers can be viewed as stimuli that promote positive feedback in the migraine loop. The smell of perfume, for example, enters the nose, producing a signal in the trigeminal nerve that is relayed to the brain stem. In most people, the brain stem damps the signal and a smaller signal is transferred harmlessly to the cortex. In migraine, however, the signal passes through to the cortex without damping, or it might even be amplified. For migraine sufferers, the signal can be intense as the feedback pathway has a low stimulus threshold, a high base signal, or is affected by a physiologically learned response. The response of the cortex also stimulates the trigeminal nerve, which produces more output and adds to the initial smell signal, increasing the overload in the brain stem.

Once this happens, a positive migraine loop takes over and no further input signal is required—the loop increases the signal with time. After this, even weak sensory inputs, such as a gentle touch on the scalp, a bright light, or normal conversation, becomes excruciating. A faint whisper is perceived as a high-pitched scream. This abnormal condition—a migraine attack—can be maintained by even slight external stimuli or normal inputs, such as the sufferer's own heartbeat pulsing through the blood vessels, which feels like hammer blows to the head.

The slightest stimulation can be a migraine trigger. Over half of people with migraines believe that the weather can cause their headaches, and there is evidence to support this view.[52] Weather triggers include it being too cold, too hot, too dry, overcast, or rainy; increased or decreased atmospheric pressure, or almost any change in conditions, may be implicated. Sunshine, or bright or fluorescent lights, can also precipitate migraines. The weather, emotional events, and similar triggers may simply provide a little extra stimulation to sensitive and hyper-responsive brain areas. It may not be the trigger that causes the problem, but rather the physiological response of the brain.

The highly developed areas of the cortex in people with migraines suggest that the brain has learned something of the process. Signals in nerves are often strengthened with use, so the progressive amplification of a response following repeated administration of a stimulus strengthens the connection.[53] Repetition of attacks may imprint the migraine physiology in the head of the sufferer. Strangely, this may mean that with each attack the body is learning how to have a migraine. Many migraine sufferers feel that whatever treatment they try, the migraine will always find a way to return. Neurologist

THE BLINK REFLEX

The importance of the feedback mechanism to those wishing to avoid migraine is highlighted by the example of blinking. Migraine patients show altered responses to stimuli that elicit blinking. The blink, or corneal reflex, is the involuntary closing and opening of the eyelids, which occurs when the outer surface of the eye is touched. It can also happen when a bright light or loud sound is experienced. Signals from the blink reflex are transmitted by the trigeminal nerve, which also carries migraine pain signals.

Generally, when a stimulus such as a loud noise is repeated, people get used it and they do not blink as much as they did the first time they heard it. In systems language, negative feedback damps the reflex response. Because of this damping, normal people show a reduced blink response to repeated stimuli, a process known as habituation. During a migraine attack, migraineurs habituate just like other people. However, migraine sufferers who are not having an attack do not habituate—they respond to each stimulus as if it were the first.[54]

This failure to habituate suggests that between migraine attacks, sufferers perceive raw signals that would normally be subject to damping at full intensity. This oversensitivity means that signals are more likely to trigger a positive feedback loop, which is implicated in migraine. A person with migraine has a hypersensitive brain and is subject to potentially disabling sensory overload.

Oliver Sacks, in his book *Migraine*, made this point clearly: it is as if the migraine is waiting, building its resources in the background, in anticipation of the opportunity to attack.[55]

Almost anything can act as a trigger, depending on the person and the current conditions. The trigger might be lack of sleep or too much sleep, or having too long an interval before drinking the next cup of coffee, allowing the first signs of caffeine withdrawal to occur. Triggers can also vary with time. In many cases, a migraine trigger merely represents a change in sensory input, which may be sufficient to overload an already hypersensitive brain. Other triggers may have a direct chemical or physiological effect.

Diet can cause migraines, particularly lack of food or specific types of food. Classical triggers include cheese, chocolate, citrus fruits, hot dogs, monosodium glutamate (MSG), aspartame, fatty foods, ice cream, caffeine withdrawal, and alcoholic drinks, especially red wine and beer.[56] Often the food in question contains an excitotoxin that can destroy brain cells. Dietary triggers affect all parts of the underlying process: they may alter the release of serotonin or adrenaline, dilate or constrict blood vessels, or stimulate the trigeminal nerves, brain stem, or brain cortex.[57]

There is a lot of confusing literature on migraine triggers—the one dependable thing about them is that they are inconsistent. Many authorities suggest keeping a diary to identify triggers or patterns in the attacks. However, interpreting the data can be difficult and the process can lead the sufferer to become unduly focused on the condition. And many migraines occur in the absence of an obvious triggering stimulus.

Some people have an attack regularly on Saturday mornings, as too much sleep at the start of the weekend can trigger an attack. Conversely, too little sleep may also result in a migraine. An alternate explanation for Saturday morning migraines is that sleeping late depletes the body of caffeine; caffeine withdrawal is a potent migraine trigger. Caffeine is abundant in the modern diet and complete avoidance is difficult for those who are sensitive. An alternative approach is to use caffeine tablets to maintain the blood levels; a dose of about 50 milligrams (mg) is sufficient to compensate for the effects of coffee withdrawal.

Migraines are often triggered by changes in lifestyle, environmental factors, or change in routine. Stress is a classic migraine trigger; however, the presence of a high level of stress can also prevent migraines. This is another explanation for Saturday morning migraines: the stress of a busy work week ends and the resulting relaxation causes a massive headache. While stressed, the person's feedback system is damped, but once the stress is relieved the damping is eased and the migraine signals are amplified. Working toward a deadline or preparing for a holiday, for example, can inhibit an attack until the stress is removed. Sadly, many a long-awaited vacation has been ruined by the sudden onset of a migraine.

Allergies as Triggers

Allergies are a source of inflammation and could often be migraine triggers. An allergy to pollen, for example, irritates the delicate lining of the nasal passages and thus the trigeminal nerve, potentially initiating an attack. However, popular descriptions of migraine allergies often include excitotoxins, such as MSG or aspartame, which produce a direct pharmacological effect. Thus, the effect might not be allergic.

There is solid evidence supporting the relationship between allergies and migraines. Allergies, especially food allergies, are often described as precipitating a migraine. A brief clinical trial with eleven patients gave excellent therapeutic results by excluding food allergens.[58] Eight patients reported substantial relief from headaches. In a study of eighty-eight children with severe migraines, eighty-two (93 percent) recovered when put on a hypoallergenic diet.[59] Several foods, rather than one individual item, affected most patients. In addition to fewer headaches, other health and behavioral benefits were reported, including reductions in abdominal pain, behavior disorders, fits, asthma, and eczema. While on the diet, most of the children became unresponsive to their usual migraine triggers. A hypoallergenic diet gave similar results in a study of children with both epilepsy and migraine.[60] Of forty-five children who had epilepsy and frequent headaches, twenty-five stopped having seizures, while a further eleven had fewer episodes. The headaches ceased along with the seizures, as well as in some children whose seizures continued.

Food allergy tests are useful for adults with migraine but diagnosing and treating allergies is difficult and time-consuming. In one study, food allergy was examined in forty-three adults with chronic migraines.[61] The study involved skin testing, elimination diets, double-blind challenges, and measurement of histamine in the blood. In thirteen subjects, a hypoallergenic diet produced a 66 percent reduction in migraine frequency, and headaches were eliminated in six patients. In terms of their response to the diet, there was a significant difference between those who had positive skin tests and those who did not: of those who had positive skin tests, eleven out of sixteen patients responded to the diet; however, only two of twenty-seven people with a negative skin test responded. Five of seven subjects who agreed to double-blind investigation experienced a migraine in response to at least one food. However, blood histamine levels, which increase with allergic reactions, increased in only three patients during the migraine-provoking challenges.

These studies suggest that allergies to food may play a role in triggering migraine attacks in some people. One method for quickly determining if allergies are involved in a particular person's migraine might be to see if a suitable antihistamine prevents an attack—if so, then it is likely that allergy is a major component. In these cases, finding and removing the allergens is the appropriate therapy. High-dose vitamin C will also help, as it is a powerful antihistamine and anti-inflammatory agent.

In some cases, linking an allergen to migraine attacks may be obvious, but in other cases it could require specialist diagnostic help. People who are unresponsive to nutritional supplements could usefully be tested for food allergens. If positive, a first step would be to try a hypoallergenic diet before considering any long-term drug therapy. Dietary modification alone may be successful.[62]

Avoiding Triggers?

Trigger factors are important, though the practical utility of investigating them is somewhat less than people often suppose. Some triggers, such as changes in atmospheric pressure, are difficult to avoid even when identified. Similarly, menstrual migraines seem to be related to changes in hormone levels, but people do not choose to be born female. Even when triggers are established and avoidable, evading them can have a detrimental effect on the person's life. Perhaps a reasonable approach is to identify the main triggers, such as excitotoxins or allergens in the diet, and remove them from the equation.

It is useful to remember that the trigger does not cause a migraine—it is just a stimulus. Other people do not respond to a migraine trigger with a headache. Moreover, a person's particular response to a trigger may vary over time: wheat may be harmless for years only to be later found to cause headaches. While migraine sufferers respond inappropriately to such stimuli, each is an individual and differs in their response. The underlying physiological controls are ineffective in migraineurs, leaving the brain in a critical condition close to overload. The trigger can be almost any stimulus that pushes the system over the edge. Avoiding obvious triggers such as food allergies may be helpful, but does not address the central problem. The problem is with the internal system and, for many, this is where the solution should be sought.

PSYCHOLOGICAL VERSUS PHYSIOLOGICAL EXPLANATIONS

There is a risk that the recurrence and resistance to treatment of migraines can be misunderstood as indicating a psychological component. This idea arises from a misunderstanding of the process. There is no "migraine personality" causing people to overachieve, suffer stress, and, as a result, have headaches. The simplest explanation is purely physiological and migraines can be explained entirely by genetics and neurology.

The notion of a psychological aspect to migraines arises from two issues. First, normal signals into the brain—for instance, from an emotional stress—are amplified in migraine to the level of pain and generate inflammation. Whether the signal is psychological or physical in origin is immaterial. By definition, an emotion is a *physiological* change in the brain, and both positive and negative emotions can cause migraine attacks. In some people, the emotional response to an affecting stimulus is to cry or laugh, but for others the stimulus is sufficient to trip the brain into signal overload and migraine.

Second, the so-called "migraine personality," rather than producing the condition, may reflect an adaptation to the illness. Migraine sufferers may make allowances for the deficits they suffer: for example, they might tend to work harder when they are not having an attack, as they know that they could be stopped in their tracks at any time. In my own case, I adapted reasonably well to anomia (the inability to remember nouns) by describing the process rather than using the name. As a student, I wrote essays on days when my brain would allow me to construct a sentence or spell a word, as an adaptation to my intermittent dyslexia. An outsider might have thought I was over-anxious to do my work, when I was just making the best of the times when I felt reasonably well.

WHY MANY MIGRAINE TREATMENTS ARE INEFFECTIVE

A simple explanation for the failure of many treatments relates to the model of migraine as a positive feedback loop. Between headaches, the responsiveness of the migraine loop is below the threshold that initiates positive feedback. A treatment that damps down the feedback signal—for example, by reducing inflammation—will lower the number of migraines, but other elements of the system may then adjust to this new condition and relax their signal damping. They do not need to damp down the signal as overload and migraine are not occurring. Gradually, the signal in the system increases over time, getting ever closer to the critical point where positive feedback is initiated. This relaxation overcomes the initial damping effect of the therapy. With time, the person returns to the point where any factor that disturbs any part of the cycle makes a migraine attack more likely.

Neurologists may ask migraine patients to switch medication every two or three months to maintain effectiveness. This may be presented as a way of compensating for the placebo effect, but changing the medication moves the damping point in the migraine cycle. Such change challenges the system's adaptation to the previous drug and may prolong the benefit, as a new physiological adaptation is required before an attack occurs. Unfortunately, with drugs there is always the risk of side effects increasing as well. Nutrients and natural remedies provide a safer way of preventing migraines.

CHAPTER 3

DIAGNOSING A MIGRAINE

Patients with migraine know precisely when and how often their headaches strike. They often come with long lists. When you have a patient with lists, you have a patient with migraine.

—SEYMOUR DIAMOND,
AUTHOR OF *CONQUERING YOUR MIGRAINE*

Headache is the name given to pain arising in the head, though this general term applies to a large number of conditions. Head pain is one of the symptoms of migraine, which is a relatively benign but disabling illness. Other conditions with similar symptoms may be life-threatening, so it is useful to be able to distinguish a dangerous head pain from a migraine or a simple headache.

TYPES OF HEADACHE

Tension Headache

Tension headache is generally mild compared to migraine, though it may be severe.[1] This form of headache can arise from muscle tension in the neck or because of stress. The pain is described as a constant pressure, as if the head were being squeezed in a vice or by a tight band around it. The pain is frequently bilateral (present on both sides of the head), although occasionally, like migraines, it can affect one side only. However, tension headaches do not share the other characteristics of migraine—pulsating pain and nausea.

Tension headaches afflict about two-thirds of adult men and over 80 percent of women.[2] These headaches often start during the teenage years and reach a maximum incidence in one's thirties. They can occur infrequently, but sometimes are chronic and happen on more than fifteen days a month.

Cluster Headache

Cluster headache is a severe localized form of migraine, of short duration and often rapid onset. The term *cluster* is used because these headaches occur in bouts of six to twelve weeks, every year or two. In some people, cluster headaches are chronic, with no gap between the clusters. Fortunately, it is relatively rare, affecting only about three in 1,000 adults.

Cluster headache is sometimes called suicide headache because of the extreme pain. Intense pain develops around one eye, once or more often each day, commonly at night. Unable to either sleep or remain lying in bed, the sufferer often paces the room, until the pain recedes thirty minutes to an hour later. Other symptoms include red and watering eyes, drooping of the eyelid on the affected side, and blocked or runny nose. Some migraine sufferers will recognize the symptoms of cluster headache, which occur in atypical migraines; the painful eye and blocked nose also occur in migraine.

Whether a headache results in someone pacing the room (as in cluster headache) or being forced to lie down (as with migraine) is sometimes used in the diagnosis. However, the two categories are closely related. My own headaches have forced me on various occasions either to pace the room or to lie immobile. Notably, with a pacing headache I cannot rest, whereas with a lying down headache I do not want to move.

Cluster headache is unusual in being more common in men than in women, which contrasts with most other forms of headache. Cluster headaches often start slightly later in life than the typical migraine, beginning in the person's twenties and continuing, sporadically, until the age of sixty or more. Anyone experiencing the onset of a cluster headache should ask their family doctor for an immediate referral to a specialist for diagnosis. However, there are few effective conventional treatments and surgery may even be recommended.[3]

As with migraines, nutritional supplementation should be the first therapy considered. The suggestions in this book, intended for migraine, may also help with cluster headaches. In particular, injections of magnesium sulfate can provide an effective treatment for cluster headaches.[4] People suffering with cluster headaches and migraines often have low blood magnesium levels and will respond to injections of magnesium sulfate, which can abort the attacks.[5] Oral supplementation with magnesium may prevent both migraines and cluster headache.

Medication Overuse Headache

People with headache often take analgesics, such as paracetamol (acetaminophen) or codeine, regularly. However, heavy use of painkillers can also cause chronic daily headaches.[6] This form of headache may be suspected if a person is having more than fifteen headache days a month.[7] Medication overuse headaches are relatively common and, like migraine, affect women more than men.[8] Nutritional supplements can be as effective as drugs in preventing migraines but do not have the side effect of causing chronic headaches.

People who have migraines often become painkiller addicts, because they self-treat with painkillers to help them deal with the pain. Unfortunately, tolerance to analgesics, especially codeine and its derivatives, builds up with time. The headaches become more frequent and the person responds by taking more painkillers. Ultimately, the person can end up with a headache that lasts all day every day. Most non-prescription analgesics, if used frequently, can lead to chronic daily headaches. The use of triptans and ergot-derived drugs for aborting a migraine attack can also cause this problem.[9] Withdrawal from the drugs may be partly effective in reducing the number of migraine attacks and chronic headaches.[10]

The World Health Organization (WHO) suggests using aspirin or ibuprofen, rather than paracetamol, for both tension and migraine headaches.[11] This may be because of the anti-inflammatory action of the aspirin-like drugs or to avoid the toxicity of paracetamol. However, nonsteroidal anti-inflammatory drugs (NSAIDs), such as aspirin, ibuprofen, and naproxen, are less likely to result in conversion of occasional migraines to chronic daily headaches. A person taking NSAIDs once or twice a day will generally be at low risk of medication overuse headache.[12] People with medication overuse headache should consider changing to NSAIDs while they recover from their dependency. In some cases, such as when the daily headache arises from NSAIDs or someone is sensitive to these drugs, this approach is inappropriate.

It is clearly important for a migraine patient to be able to distinguish a medication overuse headache from a migraine. Medication overuse headache occurs each day, usually on waking, and is persistent. Some experts think that a deciding event in the generation of medication overuse headache is the use of painkillers when the person feels an attack is imminent. However, doctors often advise migraine sufferers to take analgesics early in an attack, otherwise they may not be effective. Thus, people in this situation are in a bind. It is not at all clear when painkiller use becomes overuse, and patients need to optimize their intake to gain maximum relief without causing the headache to become chronic. Where possible, these drugs should be avoided and replaced with dietary change and supplements.

The frequency of painkiller use is important as medication overuse headache is more likely when the drug is taken every day. Higher doses taken to abort an attack are less likely to cause the problem. Guidelines for analgesic use include trying to avoid taking analgesics on more than fifteen days in a month. If frequent analgesics are necessary, use NSAIDs such as ibuprofen, since they are less likely to result in chronic daily headaches. It is recommended that codeine formulations, ergotamine, barbiturates, or the triptan medications should be limited to a maximum of about ten days each month.[13]

However, even this frequency may be too high for triptan drugs, the use of which should be limited to aborting severe attacks. Triptan drugs often lead to a relapse; in up to half the patients treated, the headache returns within a day or two. A second dose is usually effective in aborting the rebound migraine but, in some people, sec-

ond and subsequent relapses can occur. Thus, repeated use of triptans may induce medication overuse headaches.[14] Anyone using triptans to abort a migraine should be careful not to repeat the doses
too often; use a different drug for the rebound attack.

One way to minimize the risk of medication overuse headache is
to avoid using the same analgesic drug on more than two days each
week. Simply being aware that drugs can turn an occasional
migraine into a daily headache is useful. Often, people with medication overuse headache are unaware of its cause.[15] Once this
disorder has developed, early intervention is important.[16] If a particular drug is suspected, use of that drug should be stopped for a
period. Also, the offending drug should not be swapped for one
with a similar mechanism of action (for example, aspirin should not
be substituted for ibuprofen since they are both NSAIDs). Initially,
stopping a drug may make the medication overuse headache worse
and cause symptoms of withdrawal, such as sleep disturbances and
nausea.[17] It is also worth noting that medication overuse headache
tends to recur, with about four in ten patients relapsing within five
years.[18] A high relapse rate of drug overuse headache in migraine
sufferers is understandable, considering the chronic nature of the
illness.

Migraineurs are in particular danger of taking too much paracetamol (acetaminophen), which can cause liver damage. In the discomfort of a migraine attack, it is easy to forget how many and
which type of drugs have been taken. Even a small overdose of
paracetamol can be dangerous: the recommended daily maximum
dose is about 4 grams in divided doses (eight 500-mg tablets). Taking twenty or more tablets could result in liver damage.[19] The drug
inactivates glutathione, a primary cellular antioxidant in liver cells.
Acetaminophen overdose is responsible for a greater number of calls
to United States poison control centers than any other drug—over
100,000 each year.[20] Overdose causes more than 56,000 emergency
room visits, 2,600 hospitalizations, and about 458 deaths per year
in the United States Surprisingly, acetaminophen is promoted for its
safety compared to nonsteroidal analgesics, such as aspirin.

Paracetamol is one of the few poisons that have real antidotes.
Several nutritional supplements are antidotes for paracetamol poi-

soning, including L-methionine, an amino acid needed to make protein in the body. Taken prophylactically, methionine protects animals from paracetamol poisoning[21], and it has also been used as a treatment.[22] Methionine has few side effects, as it is a normal part of the diet and essential for good health. Several other dietary antioxidants, including N-acetyl-cysteine (NAC), are paracetamol antidotes.[23] Migraine patients would be well advised to supplement with NAC, methionine, alpha-lipoic acid, or liposomal glutathione, whenever they are at risk of consuming high levels of this rather dangerous drug. In general, painkillers should be used sparingly in migraine and in combination with nutritional supplements.

Chronic Daily Headache

Perhaps one in twenty adults suffers a headache on most days.[24] A chronic headache is when a person has a headache on at least fifteen days each month. Typically, chronic headaches share clinical symptoms with tension-type headaches. It is worth noting that frequent mild headaches in the front of the head may result from an eye problem, such as needing a new prescription for eyeglasses. An eye examination should be considered to exclude this cause. Clearly, medication overuse should also be ruled out as a cause of chronic headache.

Familial Hemiplegic Migraine

Familial hemiplegic migraine is a heritable form of the illness, often caused by mutations in the genes for ion channels.[25] Ion channels, such as the NMDA (*N*-methyl *D*-aspartate) receptor and its associated channel, control the flow of calcium, sodium, and other ions into nerve cells in the brain, and they are a central factor in migraines. Fortunately, hemiplegic migraine is uncommon. In the Danish population of 5.2 million people, there were only an estimated 147 cases from 44 families. There is an associated condition, which is not inherited, called sporadic hemiplegic migraine[26] and the corresponding number of cases of this sporadic form was 105, with 39 patients unable to be classified as heritable or sporadic.[27]

The symptoms of hemiplegic migraines are similar to those of standard migraines but include a reversible weakness on one side of the body, which can last for days. This may be confused with a stroke, but the effects are usually fully reversible. Other symptoms include difficulty walking, vertigo, double vision, impairment of vision or hearing, and numbness about the mouth, which can cause trouble swallowing or talking. True motor weakness and paralysis is a characteristic symptom of hemiplegic migraine. However, basilar migraine can also present with tingling or numbness.

Basilar Migraine

Basilar migraine (also known as basilar artery migraine or basilar-type migraine) is a rare form of the illness, which tends to be more common in young people. It is associated with brain stem dysfunction. (As explained earlier, the brain stem is the lower part of the brain and is continuous with the upper section of the spinal cord.) In the aura phase, strong visual disturbances may occupy the whole of both visual fields. Other symptoms include vertigo, staggering, and tingling in the limbs. In the worst cases, there can be a period of coma or paralysis, lasting up to half an hour. These preliminary symptoms are followed by a headache, which is usually at the back of the head.[28]

Basilar migraine is a serious condition that can lead to death or incapacity from stroke. Vasoconstrictor drugs, such as sumatriptan, should not be used to abort an attack, as they can increase the risk of stroke. The clinical aim of treatment is to dilate the blood vessels and restore normal blood flow to the brain stem. Basilar and hemiplegic migraines are clinically similar.[29] Doctors often use the one-sided motor weakness, or paralysis, in hemiplegic migraines to distinguish them from the basilar form.

Abdominal Migraine

Migraines are often associated with abdominal symptoms. In particular, the gut contains numerous nerves, which may partly explain the gastrointestinal symptoms in migraine. An illness called abdominal migraine occurs mainly in children, though also rarely in adults.[30] Intermittently, the child experiences nausea, vomiting, and midline abdominal pain for periods of up to three days. Children with abdominal migraine often develop migraine headaches when they are older.

CAUSES OF POTENTIALLY DANGEROUS HEADACHES

Migraines are generally considered benign, although small lesions or bright spots can occur in magnetic resonance imaging (MRI) scans of the brains of migraineurs. In a study of thirty-eight patients, these

HEADACHE/MIGRAINE TYPES	
TYPE	SYMPTOMS
Tension headache	Usually mild constant pressure, like a band around the head
Cluster headache	Excruciating pain of short duration, usually located around one red eye, nasal discharge
Medication overuse headache	Daily headache, often tension type, occurring in the mornings; caused by frequent use of painkillers
Chronic daily headache	Daily, often tension-type headache, similar to medication overuse headache
Common migraine	Intense, throbbing one-sided headache; nausea and vomiting; increased sensitivity to light, sound, smell, or movement; can last from four hours to several days
Classical migraine with aura	Warning signs (aura) occur before a migraine attack starts, such as visual disturbances, stiffness or tingling, poor balance
Familial hemiplegic migraine	Form of migraine with stroke-like symptoms; linked to genetics and runs in families
Basilar migraine	A rare, dangerous form of migraine caused by brain stem dysfunction, with similar symptoms to hemiplegic migraine
Abdominal migraine	Migraine in the gut, with vomiting, cramps, and nausea; occurs in children and less commonly in adults

minor lesions were more common in migraine with aura and basilar migraine than in migraine without aura.[31] Such changes do not appear to affect normal brain functioning. The lesions may reflect damage caused by a reduced blood supply or direct poisoning by locally released excitotoxins, such as the amino acid glutamate.

While most headaches appear to be benign, there are some that can be life-threatening. Fortunately, these are rare. The primary risk occurs in patients with moderate to severe headaches that are unusual or have abnormal features not present in the person's characteristic migraines. People who get headaches that are not typical for them, or start getting headaches later in life, should ask their physician to exclude the possibility of rare but serious conditions.

Infections

The symptoms of meningitis and encephalitis may overlap with those of migraine.[32] These include headache, stiff neck, nausea, and disturbed consciousness. Signs of fever, diarrhea, a rash, or changes in symptoms that are not common in a migraine are suggestive of infections. If there is a current risk of meningitis, such as an outbreak among university students, migraine sufferers might mistakenly delay getting treatment.

Some additional infections, mostly found in tropical regions of the world, can produce sudden severe headaches. These include dengue fever, malaria, and viral encephalitis (an infection of the brain). Travelers to these areas who suffer migraines should be aware of the need to be vigilant and not mistake the early signs of a local illness for a migraine.

Increased Pressure on the Brain

Increased pressure within the skull, with no known cause, can produce a headache. Intracranial hypertension is a rare cause of headaches and is hard to diagnose from the history alone. In adults, swelling of the optic disk at the back of the eye suggests this condition; an ophthalmologist can detect this. The condition is rare but can be caused by brain tumors.

Brain Tumors

Typically, tumors do not generate headaches until they are relatively large. However, they can raise the pressure in the brain, producing headache and other neurological signs. Since such tumors are relatively uncommon, they are not the most likely cause of head pain in patients with long-standing headache problems.[33] Tumors can cause seizures, nausea and vomiting, vision or hearing problems, inability to concentrate or find the right words, reduced patience or tolerance, and loss of inhibitions. Other symptoms include weakness of the arms, legs, or face muscles, and odd sensations in the head or hands. Since symptoms are similar to some forms of migraine, people with recurrent migraines who notice a change in their symptoms should consider informing their doctor.

Brain Hemorrhage

Subarachnoid hemorrhage, bleeding into the membranes covering the brain, can create a severe headache that comes on suddenly. Patients may describe the headache as their worst ever and also report neck stiffness. Medical advice should be sought if a severe headache occurs rapidly and the person does not have a history of similar migraine-like episodes.

Giant Cell Arteritis

A person over fifty years of age who starts to experience moderate to severe headaches may have giant cell (or temporal) arteritis, a condition of the arteries that, if left untreated, can cause serious sight loss. As in migraine, the patient may feel nausea but will have a tender scalp and feel pain on chewing or stiffness in the muscles of the jaw. The pain is usually concentrated in the temple just above the eye near to the hairline. A person with these symptoms may need urgent treatment and should see their doctor.

Glaucoma

Patients with common glaucoma do not typically have symptoms.

However, those with a rare form called angle-closure glaucoma may experience severe eye pain, nausea, blurred vision, rainbows around lights, and a red eye.[34] Symptoms may arise with a sudden increase in pressure in the eye, which becomes painful and reddened with a partially dilated and fixed pupil. The eye pain and associated headache may be intermittent and relatively mild. These symptoms are somewhat similar to cluster headaches or an atypical migraine. This form of glaucoma is an emergency and needs immediate treatment by an ophthalmologist. Left untreated, it could rapidly cause permanent loss of vision. Acute angle-closure glaucoma is rare before middle age, and a sudden onset of these symptoms later in life is a cause for concern.

GETTING AN ACCURATE DIAGNOSIS

Migraines come in various forms and the symptoms overlap with a number of diseases. It is important, therefore, to get an accurate diagnosis so the appropriate treatment can be found. A physician should be able to rule out dangerous or life-threatening conditions. The table on the following page gives a brief overview highlighting dangerous headache symptoms.

Note that head pain is a general symptom. A layperson has no direct access to specific tests, which will vary in indicating or excluding corresponding conditions. Headache is the equivalent of an engine knock in an automobile, as it can indicate problems that require further investigation to identify the cause.

The varied nature of migraine headaches is such that the physician requires the patient to provide accurate feedback on their symptoms. However, some patients may not realize that particular symptoms are associated with migraines. For instance, it may take time and repeated episodes to realize that the depression and listlessness of the prodrome is a sign of an impending attack. Moreover, one person's prodrome may be depressive, while another's feels the opposite, euphoric. Unfortunately, people may be misdiagnosed for years unless they check all their symptoms against the range of effects reported for migraine. Google your symptoms—studies suggest that Google can provide reasonably accurate diagnoses.[35]

DANGEROUS HEADACHE SYMPTOMS		
SYMPTOM	SAFE	DANGEROUS
Headache that is similar to many previous attacks	✓	
Worst headache ever		✓
Severe pain in one eye, without history of cluster headaches		✓
A headache that initially occurs later in life (over age 40 or so) with no previous headache history		✓
Blurred vision, red eye, seeing rainbows around bright lights		✓
Tingling or numbness in an arm or leg, especially one-sided		✓
Migraine with increased temperature or rash		✓
Moderate to severe headache in a child		✓
Change in usual migraine symptoms, such as tender scalp or red, watery eye		✓

Remember to check your findings with a doctor and do not (like many medical students) convince yourself that you have the last disease you read about.

Any diagnosis other than migraine (such as facial neuralgia or sinusitis) for repeated headaches, with nausea and vomiting, should be questioned.

CHAPTER 4

AVOID JUNK FOOD

I would much prefer to suffer from
the clean incision of an honest lancet
than from a sweetened poison.
—MARK TWAIN (1835–1910)

Migraine sufferers need to avoid certain food additives and to supplement their diets with protective nutrients. Flavorings in junk food may be a major cause of migraines, but this unnecessary problem can be avoided. Migraine sufferers are unusually sensitive to excitotoxins, chemical poisons that overstimulate brain cells. Many chemicals can either stimulate or dampen brain cell activity. However, excitotoxins induce brain cells to fire repeatedly, until they are exhausted and die. The brain of a migraineur is hyper-excitable and therefore more responsive to these chemicals. Excitotoxins are common in the modern diet and may contribute to brain degeneration, dementia, and epilepsy, in addition to being migraine triggers. Examples of common excitotoxins include the flavor enhancer monosodium glutamate (MSG) and the artificial sweetener aspartame.

Dietary proteins consist of linked chains of amino acids. When we eat protein foods, these long chains are broken down into individual amino acids, which are used as building blocks for our own bodies. Some amino acids act as chemical transmitters, which carry messages from one brain cell to another. Nerve cells relay messages in the form of electrical pulses stimulated by excitatory neurotransmitters. Among these are amino acids found in food, such as glutamate and aspartate, which cause nerve cells to fire more easily. By contrast, inhibitory transmitters prevent nerve cells firing; these include gamma-aminobutyric acid (GABA). The food that you eat can protect or damage the brain. Here, we explain how to modify your diet for brain health.

THE OVER-EXCITED BRAIN

Nerve cells in the brains of people with migraines are over-excitable. This sensitivity of brain cells is central to the cause of the disease. Both migraine and epilepsy share the phenomenon of increased nerve cell excitability. However, epilepsy produces a runaway excitation, in which nerve cells become synchronized. The electrical waves stimulate the brain causing epileptic seizures. In contrast, migraines involve a brief excitation followed by a wave of nerve cell inhibition, or cortical spreading depression. This damping of the signal prevents seizure in migraine attacks. The similarity between migraines and epilepsy led to a number of anti-epileptic drugs being tried for migraine, but they did not prove very effective.[1]

Magnetic resonance imaging (MRI) suggests that the depolarizing wave across the surface of the brain occurs at the same time as the migraine aura. The wave travels across the cortex of the brain at about three millimeters a minute, stimulating and then depressing the nerve cells. As the wave crosses the visual cortex, it produces the zigzag lights and other artifacts seen in the visual aura. These visual disturbances are created within the brain, though they seem to appear in the normal visual field. The visual artifacts often leave a dark spot that corresponds to the shape of the illusion, similar to the after-images produced after looking at a bright light. However, the migraine's dark spot inhibition occurs centrally within the brain, while an after-image is produced in the eye. The dark spots seen before a migraine attack are consistent with neuronal inhibition following a period of excitation.

In migraine without aura, the cortical spreading depression may stimulate areas of the brain that do not produce visual or other hallucinations. Alternately, the excitatory wave might not generate a classical aura because it is less pronounced in the visual brain areas.

However, other more subtle symptoms may be present, such as emotional depression, inability to remember words, tinnitus, or fatigue. Importantly, there may be no fundamental difference between the two types of migraine, in terms of mechanisms of action or the severity of attack. If you do not experience the visual effects of an aura, it does not mean that your migraine is less severe, as there is great variation in the presentation of the illness.

THE EFFECTS OF EXCITOTOXINS

Generally, the brain is isolated from the blood by the blood-brain barrier, which protects it from excitotoxins, many drugs, and poisons. During a migraine, however, local inflammation breaks down the blood-brain barrier, causing further local disturbances.[2] Toxins in the blood, which are normally excluded from the brain, may enter during the inflammation of a migraine attack.

Brain excitation during migraine attacks depends on local levels of excitotoxins such as glutamate. These excite the brain cells that, after a short burst of activity, are prevented from firing a signal for some time. Such inhibition may cause the cortical depression that spreads across the brain at the onset of a migraine. Glutamate can cause cortical spreading depression, resulting in a migraine attack.[3] In addition, glutamate may be involved in the pain of migraine.[4] The wave of cortical spreading depression activates the trigeminal nerve, which has branches that receive signals from the surface of the brain. In migraine, the disturbance near the brain's surface stimulates the trigeminal nerve, generating inflammation and pain[5], and these signals are returned to the top of the spinal cord at the base of the brain and, from there, back to the brain itself. This cycle of stimulation, from the brain surface through the trigeminal nerve and back to the brain's cortex, continues and increases during the migraine attack. The sensory overload and inflammation combine to cause pain.

Migraine arises from a disturbance in brain cells. The cortical electrical activity that underlies a migraine is controlled by flows of sodium, potassium, and calcium ions across the outer membrane of the brain cells. The cell membrane is a thin film of fat, which surrounds each cell and limits the transport of molecules into the cell.

Here, we are concerned with the transport of calcium into nerve cells. Calcium enters nerve cells by way of calcium channels. The NMDA (*N*-methyl *D*-aspartate) receptor, to which glutamate binds, is closely associated with one form of calcium channel. The NMDA receptor binds with glutamate or aspartate, opening the channel that allows calcium to enter the cell, making it more excitable. Thus, glutamate excites nerves cells and, by controlling calcium ion flow, the NMDA receptor acts rather like a volume control for the brain.

Women suffer migraines more than men, and one reason for this is that estrogen alters the responsiveness of NMDA receptors, can increase their number[6], and may even induce seizures at high concentration.[7] Remove the ovaries from female rodents and the number of NMDA receptors in the brain's memory circuits is reduced. Female hormones are involved in menstrual migraine and may act through their effects on the NMDA receptor.

Glutamate

In the 1960s, a phenomenon known as "Chinese restaurant syndrome" was proposed, suggesting a link between glutamate and headache. MSG is a salt form of the excitatory nerve transmitter and

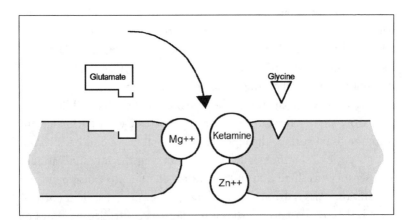

The NMDA receptor opens in the presence of glutamate, allowing calcium (Ca^{2+}) to flow into the cell. The channel is blocked by magnesium (Mg^{2+}), zinc (Zn^{2+}), and certain drugs (such as ketamine).

local hormone glutamate, which is implicated in both epilepsy and migraine. This form of glutamate occurs beyond Chinese cooking and is often added to low-quality food to improve its flavor. It is a component of stock cubes and barbecue sauce. Often its presence is hidden behind descriptions such as "hydrolyzed vegetable protein," "natural flavor," or "yeast extract." While glutamate is present in many foods at low, safe levels, MSG is a recent addition that provides an excess of glutamate. Traditional Asian cooking uses seaweed extract, which also contains glutamate. Pure MSG was not isolated and identified as a flavoring until the early years of the twentieth century, and it was patented shortly afterward.

Chinese restaurant syndrome appears to have been described first in 1968.[8] Its symptoms included burning sensations, facial pressure, and chest pain, in addition to headache. The condition was widely attributed to MSG, although research results have been conflicting. Individual responses to MSG were proportional to intake, though with considerable variation between different people.[9] Some reports suggest that Chinese restaurant syndrome is a myth, or of psychological origin.[10] However, a person suffering a new or partly understood illness is always in danger of being told it's "all in the mind." While it has long been recognized that MSG is a potential cause of migraine, clinical trials have not supported this claim consistently.[11] Nevertheless, the involvement of glutamate and related excitotoxins in migraine is not disputed.

Glutamate is the primary excitatory neurotransmitter in the brain and is a normal part of brain cell communication. In migraines, glutamate is closely associated with spreading cortical depression and stimulation of the trigeminal nerve and brain stem.[12] The resultant excitation may go unnoticed or may produce seizures, epilepsy, or migraine. In the longer term, glutamate may contribute to brain degeneration and dementia.

Most of the time, the blood-brain barrier protects the brain from toxins in the blood. The barrier is formed from tightly packed cells in the blood vessels of the brain. This tight packing hinders substances in the bloodstream from entering brain tissues. Glutamate is often assumed safe in the diet, presumably because the blood-brain barrier prevents toxicity to the brain. But assuming the brain is protected from excitotoxins in the diet may be an unfortunate oversimplification. The blood-brain barrier occasionally may not be intact, allowing poisons to breach the brain's defenses.[13] This breakdown may be important both in migraine and in degenerative brain diseases, such as dementia.

Moreover, not all of the brain is protected in this way. Near the center of the brain, the hypothalamus, which is involved in hormone and appetite regulation, is directly affected by glutamate in the bloodstream. The high and increasing incidence of obesity in recent decades could be a result of glutamate and other excitotoxins destroying nerve cells in the hypothalamus, including those involved in the control of eating. Scientists have experimented on young rats to find out what happens if they are fed glutamate.[14] In animals, two characteristics of glutamate toxicity are voracious eating and lowered growth hormone levels. MSG, in amounts only a little greater than found in human food, can damage the hypothalamus in animals, making them short, stunted, and fat. Scientists regularly use glutamate to create fat rats for experimentation. Recently, scientists have warned that similar MSG effects may be occurring in humans.[15]

There are many possible explanations for the conflicting findings with respect to Chinese restaurant syndrome. There is large individual variation and people have differing propensities for migraine headaches. Furthermore, migraineurs have a wide range of responses to dissimilar triggers. The effects of MSG are not consistently confirmed in clinical trials, but this could reflect the bias introduced when any substance has associated economic profit. However, migraineurs should avoid glutamate despite somewhat variable evidence. Inflammation in the brain and surrounding blood vessels might lead the blood-brain barrier to leak, allowing excitotoxins to enter the brain. The blood-brain barrier may already be compromised in people with a propensity to migraine headaches.[16] Moreover, during a migraine attack, the blood-brain barrier may not function properly.[17] Disturbances to the blood-brain barrier may even be an underlying cause of migraine.[18]

When the blood-brain barrier fails, excitotoxins and other chemicals can enter the brain, causing local inflammation and damage. Lesions in the white matter of the brain have been linked to damage in small blood vessels.[19] While the brain's gray matter contains large numbers of nerve cell bodies, white matter consists largely of long thin projections that transmit signals to and from nerve cells, rather like electrical cables. In migraine sufferers, small areas of white matter may be damaged and can appear as bright spots in magnetic resonance images.[20] Such lesions, rather than being a result of the migraine, may predispose to the condition, as they are associated with a local breakdown of the blood-brain barrier.

These areas of damage may be caused by a reduced blood supply or the release of excitotoxins. In high concentration, the excitatory amino acids glutamate and aspartate kill brain cells, and glutamate is present in the areas of the brain associated with migraine.[21] Compared with normal people, those with migraine may have higher levels of excitatory amino acids, including glutamate and aspartate, in both blood[22] and brain.[23] The levels of neurotransmitters in the brains of migraineurs differ from normal controls[24], and glutamate increases during a migraine attack.[25] However, the evidence is neither complete nor consistent.[26]

People who suffer from migraines are at specific risk from excitotoxins. If local inflammation, or lack of oxygen, becomes extreme, brain cells may be damaged when large amounts of glutamate are released.[27] Brain cells release glutamate when stressed in this way. Extreme migraine can lead to a form of stroke, which has generally been assumed to be caused by vascular disease or clotting. Reduced blood supply to areas of the brain is characteristic of migraine. Equally, however, the stroke effects could result from the subsequent massive release of glutamate, which damages or kills brain cells. In migraine patients, brain abnormalities that can be interpreted as stroke may be a result of local excitotoxin damage. It is, therefore, particularly advisable for people with migraines to avoid dietary excitotoxins.

"Sweet Poison"

Another excitotoxin that is important to migraine sufferers is L-aspartyl-L-phenylalanine-1-methyl ester, better known as aspartame. Aspartame is a popular artificial sweetener that is about 180 times sweeter than table sugar. It is used extensively in soft drinks and foods to the point where it is difficult to exclude from the diet unless one is extremely vigilant. Aspartame is a migraine trigger.[28]

Aspartame is relatively unstable and tends to break down spontaneously, during storage of foods or beverages. When broken down, aspartame can release methanol (wood alcohol), formaldehyde, and two amino acids, aspartate and phenylalanine. About one-tenth of the aspartame that is consumed breaks down to generate methanol in the gut, which is absorbed and converted to formaldehyde and then formic acid. Formaldehyde, which is used in embalming fluid, cross-links tissues, including DNA, and may cause cancer. About half the mass of ingested aspartame is released as an essential amino acid called phenylalanine. In people with phenylketonuria, a hereditary disease, this substance can cause mental retardation and seizures. Clearly, these people should avoid foods containing aspartame.

As it breaks down, aspartame also produces the excitotoxin aspartate, and resultant high blood levels[29] can damage the brain.[30] Proponents of aspartame suggest that the release of aspartate is not harmful in humans. While it causes damage to the brains of animals, they suggest that the blood-brain barrier and species differences render it safe for human use.[31] However, other evidence suggests that when methanol is given along with either aspartate or glutamate, it facilitates penetration of nervous tissue by the amino acids.[32]

The most frequently reported side effect of aspartame is headache. The medical literature contains reports of people getting migraines after chewing sugarless gum[33], suggesting that even a low intake of aspartame could cause a problem for some people. The phenomenon could be related to dose; for example, additional aspartame is reported to have increased the severity of aspartame migraine in two patients.[34] In one case study, a 31-year-old woman thought her migraines were caused by consuming aspartame tablets (1.0–1.5 grams per day) and soft drinks containing aspartame.[35] When she stopped the diet drinks and aspartame, her headaches disappeared in ten days. Following this, she tested the idea by drinking a 500-mg aspartame solution, which produced a migraine in ninety minutes. The test was repeated using saccharin or sugar, neither of which resulted in headaches.

The use of aspartame as a food additive has been sanctioned by the U.S. Food and Drug Administration (FDA) and other government health organizations. Despite claims for its safety[36], aspartame has been linked to diseases such as cancer, brain lesions, and mental disorders.[37] Psychiatrist Ralph G. Walton, M.D., of Northeastern Ohio University, examined bias in aspartame research by reviewing 166 studies in the peer-reviewed medical literature, noting the outcome and the source of funding.[38] The aspartame industry funded seventy-four of the studies, and ninety-two were independent. All of the industry-funded papers confirmed aspartame's safety and none reported any health problems. By comparison, only seven (7.6 percent) of the independent studies reported that aspartame was safe; the remaining studies suggested an adverse reaction. Dr. Walton's examination provides a strong indication of bias in the medical literature.

Following the introduction of aspartame as a food additive, a large number of complaints about the side effects of aspartame were submitted to the FDA.[39] By 1996, the number of official complaints submitted for headache as a side effect of aspartame was 1,847 (19 percent of the total). As we have seen, headache is only one symptom

TOP TEN COMPLAINTS TO THE FDA ABOUT ASPARTAME	
SYMPTOM	NUMBER OF COMPLAINTS
1. Headache	1,847
2. Dizziness or poor equilibrium	735
3. Mood change	656
4. Vomiting/nausea	647
5. Abdominal pain and cramps	483
6. Change in vision	362
7. Diarrhea	330
8. Seizures and convulsions	290
9. Memory loss	255
10. Fatigue/weakness	242

of migraine. When we consider the top ten aspartame complaints, the picture is disconcerting. Apart from the abdominal complaints, seizures, and diarrhea (which are rare migraine effects, but do occur), the list is a description of migraine symptoms. Moreover, this list of symptoms might be expected from ingesting an excitotoxin.

PROTECTING THE BRAIN

To help prevent migraines, avoid excitotoxins. Excitotoxins are implicated in migraines because of the way they affect NMDA receptors. These receptors, found on the surface of nerve cells in the brain, interact with glutamate and aspartate. When the receptors are activated, a channel is opened in the cell membrane, allowing calcium to enter the cell. The calcium flow through the channel may influence learning and memory, and it also plays a central role in migraine, brain degeneration, and nerve cell death.

Overstimulation of the NMDA receptor is dangerous to cells, so the brain has many regulatory processes to try to avoid excitotoxicity. The NMDA receptor depends not only on the presence of glutamate or aspartate, but needs the presence of the amino acids glycine or serine for proper function. Also, opening the ion channel depends on the voltage difference across the cell wall.

Since excitotoxicity is damaging to the brain, drugs that act on the NMDA receptor have been developed, including amantadine, dextromethorphan, dextrorphan, ketobemidone, memantine, and tramadol. Most of these drugs work by blocking the channel and stopping it from responding to glutamate. While this would appear to offer fantastic potential for preventing migraines and brain damage, there are drawbacks. NMDA receptor antagonists, as they are called, though sometimes used as anesthetics, are not widely available. At higher doses, they have hallucinogenic properties and several (ketamine, nitrous oxide, and PCP or phencyclidine) are recreational drugs. In addition to being involved in migraines, NMDA receptors are directly implicated in depression[45] and degenerative brain diseases. Ketamine has been shown to give rapid and lasting relief from depression.[46] Depression is a symptom of migraine, but only accounts for part of the debility it causes.

PLACEBO OR EXCITOTOXIN?

In modern medical research, a placebo is assumed to be a substance that has no physiological effect. Researchers use placebos to show that a new drug is more effective than a sham treatment. This may be preferred by drug companies as it is a less demanding test than showing the new drug could outperform an older, less expensive drug. A placebo can be anything the researcher decides is inert. Surprisingly, many medical papers fail to state what substance was used as a placebo or to give the authors' reasons for believing it has no biological effect. Notably, in many migraine studies, the placebo can be an excitotoxin or migraine trigger.

Dr. Frederick Strong, a researcher in Brazil, noticed that, in six studies, almost one-fifth of diet-sensitive migraine patients reported getting headaches from the placebo.[40] In these studies, the placebos were concealed in gelatin capsules. Gelatin is a form of collagen jelly obtained from animal bones and skin; it contains partially hydrolyzed animal proteins. As a migraine sufferer himself, the researcher knew that hydrolyzed vegetable protein could cause migraines, and wondered whether the gelatin capsules could be having a similar effect.[41] He found that the so-called placebo capsules may cause migraines, as they contained known triggers (excitotoxins). Patients might have expected researchers to realize that using placebos that release excitotoxins could induce migraine headaches.

In some studies of monosodium glutamate (MSG) as a migraine trigger, the placebo control was aspartame! Since aspartame is a migraine trigger releasing the excitotoxin aspartate, these studies compare the difference between two excitotoxins, glutamate and aspartate.[42] To confuse matters further, aspartame was used as a masking sweetener for both the MSG and the placebo. The inappropriate use of placebos is contaminating the medical literature, compromising independent evaluation, and delaying the scientific process.

Another way the use of inappropriate placebos can confound the results of an experiment is if the researchers choose a placebo that is able to prevent migraines. Later, we will see that riboflavin (vitamin B$_2$) is an effective migraine preventative. One study attempted to test the effectiveness of a combination of riboflavin, magnesium, and the herb feverfew, each of which can prevent migraines.[43] Since riboflavin has a distinctive yellow color, the researchers decided to use a low dose of it as a placebo. The authors found no significant differences between the low-dose riboflavin and the combination therapy. However, they noted that both groups showed significant improvement from their baseline migraine frequency. These results can easily be explained: the maximum amount of riboflavin that can be absorbed from a single dose is about 27 milligrams[44], so the placebo was likely to be as effective as the higher-dose treatment.

It is easy to see that if the researchers had not described what was in their placebos, the trials could have been misinterpreted. Such trials can be a gift to anyone wanting to bias results: a shrewd choice of placebo can make a drug therapy seem effective or a vitamin therapy ineffective, when the opposite may be true.

There are NMDA modulators that can stabilize the receptors and channels without complete blockade of glutamate and aspartate activity. Such modulators may be useful in controlling migraine, mood disorders such as severe depression[47], and degenerative brain disease. Notably, magnesium has two direct effects on the NMDA receptors. It physically blocks the NMDA channel, though this action depends on the voltage across the cell membrane—at more positive voltages, it can increase the cell's responsiveness. Magnesium supplements have also been reported to produce rapid recovery from major depression.[48] Zinc also blocks the NMDA receptors and, like magnesium, is reported to have antidepressive properties.[49] As explained later, magnesium, zinc, and other nutrients offer a safe approach to the treatment of migraine.

Antioxidants

Antioxidant nutrients protect the brain and are beneficial in migraine. NMDA receptors are regulated by the local level of antioxidants, which prevent oxidation damage. Oxidation refers to the loss of electrons, which makes a molecule less stable, creating damaging free radicals that attempt to "steal" electrons from other molecules. The opposite, reduction, is the gain of electrons, which returns the molecule to a more stable state.

The behavior of an NMDA receptor is regulated by oxidants. A section of the protein of the NMDA receptor, called the redox modulatory site, responds to oxidation. (*Redox* is short for reduction-oxidation.) The redox site is affected by changes in the level of antioxidants: antioxidants increase NMDA channel activity, oxidants depress the activity.[50] This means that antioxidants can influence NMDA receptors without directly affecting the action of glutamate or drugs.[51]

Generally, antioxidants protect brain cells by mopping up free radicals, which are harmful to cells. However, at the NMDA redox site, oxidants may make glutamate less damaging to brain cells.[52] The action of antioxidants on NMDA receptors is not straightforward: some, such as vitamin C, inhibit NMDA receptors, while others potentiate them.[53] Vitamin C inhibits binding of glutamate to the NMDA receptor complex. One explanation for this complex behavior is that damage and inflammation involve free radicals and oxidation. When healthy, the brain is in a relatively reducing state, with fewer damaging free radicals and oxidation. In this state, the brain cells are free to respond to glutamate. In the presence of overstimulation or inflammation, the local tissue becomes more oxidizing. This oxidation may inhibit the NMDA receptor, preventing damaging overstimulation of the cell.

Antioxidants can also block the toxic effects of excitotoxins in the brain indirectly. The toxicity of glutamate in the brain depends on nitric oxide.[54] Nitric oxide, in addition to promoting inflammation, expands local blood vessels and can be a cause of headache. Excess glutamate results in a local accumulation of dangerous free radicals, causing damage to nerve cells.[55] As the cells' energy and antioxidant production are disturbed, they become increasingly sensitive to stress and inflammation. Sensitivity to stress, signal overload, and a propensity for inflammation are characteristics of migraines. For this reason, antioxidant supplements such as vitamin C may provide a level of protection against the stresses of migraine and help recovery.

Avoid Brain-Destroying Additives

People with migraines should avoid any food containing high levels of glutamate and aspartate. Artificial sweeteners and foods containing MSG may be the cause of numerous unnecessary migraine headaches. However, aspartame has become abundant in many packaged foods, beverages, and candies. This is compounded by the occurrence of high levels of glutamate in many processed foods. A migraineur who eats Chinese food and a bag of potato chips for lunch, followed by a low-calorie pudding washed down with a diet cola, might consume gram levels of excitotoxins.

The best advice for migraine sufferers is to avoid junk food. Keep away from MSG, stock cubes, barbecue sauce, flavor enhancers, hydrolyzed vegetable protein, natural flavors, and yeast extract. You should also avoid artificial sweeteners, as the benefit in terms of lower calories is more than offset by the potential to cause headaches. If you inadvertently eat excitotoxins, magnesium and zinc supplements will protect the brain. Antioxidant vitamins and supplements can provide additional protection. In addition to lowering the frequency of migraines and keeping your brain healthy, these minor changes will provide a more interesting and rewarding diet.

CHAPTER 5

PREVENTING A MIGRAINE
WITH NUTRITION

*A migraine is like a tornado. It attacks fast, usually
without warning, and wreaks havoc regardless of
what's going on in your life at that moment.*
—STEPHEN SILBERSTEIN, DIRECTOR OF THE
COMPREHENSIVE HEADACHE CENTER,
THOMAS JEFFERSON UNIVERSITY, PHILADELPHIA

For prevention of migraines, medicine based on nutritional supplements is at least as effective as the most powerful drugs. Unfortunately, this is not as strong a claim as it might appear, because
migraine drugs are limited in their effectiveness: they work in about
half the patients who take them. Even then, they are not foolproof,
as typically they prevent only about half the migraine attacks. Then,
the benefit is only partial relief. This poor performance is because
when the drugs were developed, the underlying pathology of the illness was not well understood, so drugs for other conditions have
been employed. In addition, anti-migraine medications have potentially serious side effects.

Migraine headaches are difficult to control. Anti-epileptic drugs
have occasionally proved useful, as they help prevent cortical spreading depression. Similarly, antidepressants and drugs for high blood
pressure can prevent some migraines. However, if drugs are to be
used, the correct prescription for any particular patient has to be
determined by trial and error. Even after this has been done, the drug
may work for only a short period before the migraines find a way

STAMP COLLECTING OR SCIENCE?

Current medical research makes little reference to evolution. This is unfortunate, as biology (of which medicine is an applied branch) is hard to understand without an evolutionary perspective. Evolution provides a framework for understanding physiology, biochemistry, and disease, and offers a more strategic viewpoint than is usual in current genetic and social medicine.

Substances from animals, plants, fungi, and other organisms are vital for human health and well-being. Without vitamins, obtained from plants and bacteria, we would not survive. Additionally, many of our most powerful or useful drugs come from plants, including morphine, digitalis, cocaine, taxol, cannabis, caffeine, L-dopa, nicotine, and quinine. The fact that plants offer such wealth is neither accident nor magic. Plants evolved as stationary organisms, gaining their energy from sunlight. Because they don't move, they have to manufacture their essential chemicals from substances about them. A plant is therefore a complex biochemical factory. Animals, by contrast, can roam to find food: they do not need to synthesize all their own chemicals, as the plants they eat can provide what they need.

As a result of their evolutionary path, animals have benefited from the internal chemical machinery of plants. But why do plants happen to produce the very substances animals need? One reason is that plants and animals share common ancestors, so much of their core biochemistry is the same. For example, almost all animals and plants produce vitamin C at high levels, as a water-soluble antioxidant. Humans, however, do not have this ability; at some stage during evolution, our ancestors lost a gene involved in the synthesis of vitamin C. Presumably, they did this at a time when they were able to consume lots of vitamin C-rich plant material. Consequently, they became dependent on vitamin C from plants, without which people get scurvy and ultimately die.

Evolution causes the health of animals to depend critically

on substances derived from the diet. If such nutrition is not available, the animal's growth and well-being will suffer. Nutritional deprivation will result in chronic disease. Modern medicine, however, while paying lip service to nutritional factors, seems to consider people as more likely to be drug-deficient than nutrient-deficient.

Medicine has lost touch with its roots in biological science. It is becoming a technology, based on trial-and-error developments, as opposed to fundamental research. The differences between science and technology are blurred by the current fashion for social and genetic medicine. Modern medicine is becoming more like stamp collecting than science. A common putdown in medicine is "that's only theoretical." Similar digs are encountered in relation to animal studies, experimental results, or physiological systems. Such statements are misguided: in science, there is nothing more important than theory and experimentation.

around it. As one pathological pathway for the attack is inhibited, the migraine mechanism adjusts to follow an alternative route.

With increasing knowledge, targeted treatment of migraine is gradually becoming available. New pharmaceutical approaches include preventing inflammation and targeting NMDA (N-methyl D-aspartate) channels in nerve cells. Similar or greater effects can be achieved using nutritional treatments, which avoid the side effects and costs associated with conventional drugs.

DIET AND MIGRAINE PREVENTION

Low-Carbohydrate Diet

Diet influences migraine and related disorders, such as epilepsy. Migraineurs sometimes discover this by accident; for example, when trying a low-carbohydrate diet to lose weight, they find they have fewer headaches. One well-known "low-carb" diet was made popular by Robert Atkins, M.D., an orthomolecular physician.[1] Low-carbohydrate diets have a long history and Atkins' approach was a development of the Banting diet, named after William Banting, one of the first to develop the idea in the nineteenth century.[2]

Carbohydrates provide glucose, the brain's main energy source. When glucose is limited, the liver breaks down fatty acids to produce ketone bodies, an alternative energy supply for the brain. The state of being short of glucose, so that high levels of ketones are formed, is called ketosis. Diets that are very low in carbohydrates are keto-genic—they induce the production of ketones. In the 1920s, it was known that fasting for one to three weeks could prevent seizures for many subsequent weeks. As a result, ketosis and dietary restriction were used as effective treatments for epilepsy for nearly a century.

In 1938, the drug phenytoin was found to control seizures with-out the sedative effects of the earlier barbiturate anticonvulsant pheno-barbital.[3] As it is more convenient—not to mention more profitable —to take a pill than to fast or stick to a low-carbohydrate diet, the ketogenic diet fell out of favor and the chance of achieving a greater understanding of epilepsy was lost. In some people, however, epi-lepsy is resistant to drugs and the ketogenic diet may be the most appropriate therapy. Notably, the ketogenic diet is still used as an anti-epileptic treatment in children when seizures are drug resistant.[4]

In the mid-1990s, the ketogenic diet regained popularity, partly because of the film *First Do No Harm* (1997) starring Meryl Streep, which was based on the true story of a child with epilepsy. The direc-tor, Jim Abrahams, had a son with severe epilepsy, which was even-tually treated by the diet. After his son's experience, Abrahams was amazed that the diet was not in widespread use and set up a foun-dation to publicize it and fund research. When patients are forced to investigate the causes of an illness in order to develop, or redis-cover, old treatments, it brings into question the organization and effectiveness of modern "scientific" medicine.

A recent Cochrane review of the ketogenic diet reported that there was "no reliable evidence from randomized, controlled trials to sup-port the use of ketogenic diets for people with epilepsy."[5] (The Cochrane Collaboration provides selective reviews of medicine for health-care professionals.) In fact, there were no randomized, controlled trials at all, supportive or otherwise. The authors suggested that the diet was a "possible option" in the treatment of intractable epilepsy—in other words, if no drugs were effective in a particular case, the diet may be tried. This response is typical of so-called evidence-based medicine, in which only selective evidence is considered. In their view, only randomized trials provide reliable evidence. However, the review noted that there were "large observational studies, some prospective, suggesting an effect on seizures." Considering the devastating effect of seizures, a change in diet that has been reported effective in studies spanning nearly a century might be considered worthy of respect. The reason for the lack of what the review termed "reliable" evidence is simply that medical science has failed to perform the required studies. Often authors writing from a selective "evidence-based" viewpoint, which includes many Cochrane reviewers, fail to appreciate that, unlike drugs, dietary change can provide benefit with little risk.

In 2008, a randomized trial of the diet showed positive results in epilepsy.[6] The study involved 145 children, 73 on the ketogenic diet and 72 controls, and ran for three months. In the diet group, 38 percent had half their previous number of seizures, compared with 6 percent of controls; 7 percent of those on the diet had less than one-tenth as many seizures, whereas no controls achieved this reduction. Side effects included constipation, vomiting, lack of energy, and hunger. These children had already failed to respond to at least two anti-epileptic drugs, so the positive response is of particular importance to children with drug-resistant epilepsy or migraines.

The National Institute for Clinical Excellence (NICE), in the United Kingdom, states that the ketogenic diet "should not be recommended for adults with epilepsy."[7] But they did suggest it might be used with children. NICE claims, like Cochrane, that the basis of their recommendation is the lack of randomized clinical trials. Assessing the effects of ketogenic diets on seizures, they reported twenty studies (from the Cochrane review) that suggested a potential beneficial effect, which NICE interpreted as indicating that randomized controlled trials were needed. Presumably, NICE intends that patients who do not respond to drugs must remain untreated while they wait the years needed to complete the clinical trials. So far, such patients would have waited eight decades for the research to be conducted! The dissenting view is that the ketogenic diet shows promise in adult epilepsy.[8] Adults who have the information often choose to try the diet.

No one disputes that diet affects migraines. The ketogenic diet has often been tried as a means of preventing intractable migraine, but little has been published in the medical literature. Migraine and epilepsy share an underlying pathology and, if a ketogenic diet is effective for epilepsy, it may provide relief for migraine sufferers.[9] Notably, ketogenic diets are reported to modify levels of glutamate and inhibitory amino acids in the brain; this effect could provide a direct mechanism to explain the benefit.[10]

One caution for migraineurs undertaking a low-carbohydrate diet is that it may make them more susceptible to excitotoxic migraine triggers, because abundant glucose provides some protection against excitotoxins.[11] Brain cells are more sensitive to excitotoxins, such as aspartame or MSG, when glucose is in short supply. For this reason, people embarking on a low-carb diet might consider supplementing with magnesium, multivitamins and minerals, and antioxidants, which could also help overcome the potential for induced nutritional deficiency.

If other treatments do not work for someone with migraines, or if the person needs to lose weight, a low-carbohydrate diet might be considered. However, it would not be sensible to keep to a strict low-carb diet during a migraine attack. The urge for sweet food that often precedes the attack may be the brain's way of loading with carbohydrates as a protection from excitotoxins. Eating food high in carbohydrates, such as a handful of dried fruit, is occasionally effective in preventing my migraine attacks.

The Gerson Diet

Dr. Max Gerson's diet is widely used in unconventional cancer therapy. However, Dr. Gerson seems to have become interested in diet and health because of his migraine headaches. By eliminating particular foods from his diet, he was apparently able to become headache free. Prescribing his anti-migraine diet to patients, he found that they reported other conditions, such as tuberculosis, were improved.

The Gerson anti-cancer diet involves raw, vegan food and fresh organic juices. He also suggested providing hydrogen peroxide and supplements such as vitamin C. While Dr. Gerson is often ridiculed for suggesting coffee enemas, his diet is close to the more recent redox therapy diet.[12] Dr. Gerson originally developed his diet in the 1920s and knowledge of nutrition has increased greatly since that time. However, the Gerson approach may be an effective cancer therapy.[13] The main difference from redox therapy is Dr. Gerson's emphasis on juicing, which releases nutrients from fruits and vegetables, but may be counterproductive, as it potentially provides the cancer cells with nutrients that are essential for tumor growth.

Dr. Gerson's anti-migraine diet was found to be useful for a range of health conditions, such as diabetes and arthritis. This illustrates the main side effect with nutritionally based approaches to migraines—greatly improved general health and a reduction in illness and disease. These benefits are in addition to the direct improvement in migraine relief, and they contrast with the negative, health-draining side effects of conventional drug therapies.

CONTROLLING ALLERGIES

If your migraines occur during the hay fever season, seem to respond to anti-histamines, or are intractable to other treatments, consider allergies as a cause. Food allergies should also be investigated, along with excitotoxins and other potential migraine triggers. As described earlier, food sensitivity and other allergies have long been associated with migraines, though this area is somewhat controversial. One reason for this controversy is that rigorous determination of food and other allergies is a complex and rather difficult process.[14] A total elimination diet may be required, which is not easy to undertake or manage. Skin testing is a simpler process and may also be effective.[15]

For those suffering with a food allergy, removing the offending substances from the diet should provide relief. If this is impractical, one approach is to follow the lead of Robert Cathcart, M.D., and try dynamic flow-level doses of vitamin C daily.[16] Dynamic flow requires several grams of vitamin C each day, taken in divided doses.

Dr. Cathcart was known for his work on vitamin C and infections, but allergies were also a major area of interest to him. One of the reasons why he became interested in vitamin C was its effectiveness in stopping the allergies he had suffered with for many years. (I had the great pleasure of working with him on the dynamic flow of vitamin C.) Vitamin C is a potent anti-histamine and Dr. Cathcart routinely used massive oral doses to combat allergies in patients.

ESSENTIAL NUTRIENTS

Vitamins and minerals can play a key role preventing migraines. For example, both riboflavin (vitamin B_2) and magnesium can prevent migraines, with effects approximating the most effective drugs. These nutrients are essential to the diet and have few side effects.

Magnesium and Zinc

The protective benefits of magnesium and zinc make them essential supplements for anyone with migraines. Both zinc and magnesium are lower in hair samples from migraineurs.[17] The combination of magnesium and zinc is the first line of defense against migraine attacks, as it inhibits the action of excitotoxins at the NMDA receptor.[18] For this reason, magnesium and zinc can be considered together in the prevention of migraines. They can help protect the brain from excitotoxins and other migraine-related insults.

Magnesium

Magnesium interferes with two of the main mechanisms underlying migraine: it blocks the glutamate (NMDA) receptors and inhibits nitric oxide synthesis and release. In addition, magnesium is a smooth muscle relaxant and may stabilize vulnerable blood vessels. The importance of magnesium for people with migraine headaches is well established through clinical and experimental studies.[19] People with migraines have low magnesium levels in their cells, saliva, and blood[20], and brain levels of magnesium are low during an attack.[21]

There are excellent reasons for believing magnesium may prevent migraine attacks. When injected, magnesium sulfate rapidly aborts a full-blown migraine. However, the amount absorbed in oral doses is inadequate to end an established migraine. Despite this, a first step in migraine therapy should be to make sure the migraineur is not magnesium deficient and has a high oral intake. Oral magnesium supplements can increase intracellular magnesium levels, which compensates for the common deficiency that can make brain cells more excitable and bring on a migraine attack.[22]

Supplementation with magnesium (600 mg a day) has been shown to reduce the number of migraine headaches. In one study, eighty-one migraine patients, 18–65 years old, had an average of 3.6 attacks each month.[23] For twelve weeks, they received either a placebo or 600 mg of magnesium each day. Between weeks nine and twelve, the attack frequency in the magnesium group was significantly lowered below the baseline. Those taking magnesium had fewer days with migraines and required less medication to relieve their acute symptoms. Adverse effects included diarrhea and stomach irritation; these can be prevented by taking the magnesium in several doses throughout the day or by lowering the amount taken.

Conversely, a placebo-controlled study found that magnesium (485 mg per day) did not reduce the frequency of migraine headaches.[24] It is possible that this study used a poorly absorbed or contaminated form. In another trial, researchers found that oral magnesium oxide reduced headache frequency over the sixteen-week intervention period in children with migraines. The use of magnesium oxide in this study is rather surprising, since this form is poorly absorbed when taken orally.[25] Perhaps these children were deficient and the small amount of magnesium absorbed was corrective.

A new drug called memantine has a mechanism of action similar to that of magnesium. Indeed, the drug may have resulted from a search for a patentable substance to mimic magnesium. Memantine was the first drug aimed at preventing Alzheimer's disease by blocking NMDA receptors.[26] Its aim is to block excitotoxin damage to nerve cells and thus prevent dementia from progressing. Memantine is currently being proposed as a preventative treatment for migraine[27] and trial results suggest its effectiveness is similar to that of magnesium supplements.[28] Memantine restores function in brain cells depleted of magnesium.[29] However, as a migraine treatment, it may simply compensate for a chronic nutritional deficiency of magnesium in a less-than-obvious way. Memantine appears to be an expensive replacement for magnesium but with side effects, including headache, vomiting, drowsiness, confusion, dizziness, insomnia, agitation, hallucinations, anxiety, and cystitis.

While most adults are deficient in magnesium intake, individual requirements vary. Typically, adults should have an intake of 300–400 mg of elemental magnesium each day. Migraineurs may need more, perhaps as high as 600–700 mg daily. This is below the minimum level at which adverse effects are reported. However, magnesium acts as a laxative and migraineurs need to ensure that their particular tolerance is not exceeded. Note that these values refer to the weight of the metal or element. Many supplements quote the total weight of the salt form; for example, 200 mg of magnesium citrate may be the total weight of both the magnesium and citrate combined. Make sure you check the weight of *elemental* magnesium in the supplement.

Migraineurs need to be careful in selecting magnesium supplements, because many will have no effect on migraines or might even make the illness worse. You may have tried magnesium and found it did not work—the likely reason is that you used the wrong form. For example, the common oxide form is barely absorbed (about 1 percent) when taken orally, so it cannot be expected to prevent migraines. Low-cost supplements often contain magnesium oxide; the rule of thumb is to read the label and avoid the oxide form.

Magnesium aspartate is a common, easily absorbed form, but unfortunately the magnesium is bound to the excitotoxic amino acid aspartate, which can instigate migraine attacks. Migraine sufferers should therefore avoid this form of magnesium. Supplements of magnesium glutamate, another excitotoxic form, are fortunately rare. However, other easily absorbed forms of magnesium may contain glutamate or aspartate, completely negating any beneficial effects. Some absorbable forms of magnesium are described as "magnesium amino acid chelate" or simply "magnesium chelate," but the particular amino acid is not named. These terms should generate suspicion. If you take this form, you may be taking a migraine-triggering excitotoxin along with your magnesium. Excitotoxins can contaminate other apparently innocuous supplements, such as magnesium citrate. A purchaser might expect a magnesium citrate supplement to consist of magnesium bound to citric acid, which is found in many "citrus" fruits, such as oranges, lemons, and limes. However, when used as a food additive, citric acid is listed as frequently containing excitotoxins[30] and may be contaminated with unwelcome substances. Again, it is crucial to read the label.

Do not despair! Several forms of magnesium supplement absorb well and can be taken with benefit. Look for supplements containing magnesium chloride, ascorbate, glycinate, gluconate, lactate, malate, or orotate. (People who are lactate intolerant should avoid the lactate form.) I would normally recommend magnesium ascorbate, chloride, or perhaps malate. With magnesium ascorbate, you get extra vitamin C "free" with your magnesium. However, it is important to avoid supplements containing mixtures of calcium and magnesium, as they are chemically similar and compete for absorption into the body. Also, high plasma levels of calcium relative to magnesium are characteristic of migraine.[31]

Perhaps the optimal way of delivering magnesium for migraine would be in the form of liposomes. Liposomes are microscopic spheres of fat (phospholipid) containing a nutrient or a drug. In this form, an oral preparation might be used to abort a migraine with no side effects. Unfortunately, there is a patent on liposomal magnesium for use in migraine and brain injury, which currently restricts its production.[32]

Some people bathe in Epsom salts, a common name for magnesium sulfate. Magnesium may be absorbed through the skin, so adding Epsom salts to bathwater can increase levels in the body.[33] Migraineurs report that bathing in Epsom salt water can relieve migraine attacks. Given the low oral absorption of magnesium, adding Epsom salts to the bath may be a useful preventative technique for migraine sufferers.

Zinc

Migraine sufferers should avoid zinc deficiency. Like magnesium, zinc inhibits NMDA receptors,[34] but there may be variability over regions of the brain.[35] There do not appear to be any clinical trials on zinc supplementation for migraines, either alone or in combination with magnesium. Zinc may be released from nerve cells during an epileptic attack,[36] and zinc deficiency increases susceptibility to epileptic attacks.[37] Zinc may be a factor in nerve damage, both in epilepsy and when the brain lacks oxygen in migraine.[38]

Zinc intake affects copper levels. Several trigger factors for migraine, such as citrus fruits and chocolate, contain or increase absorption of copper.[39] Copper intrauterine contraceptive devices (IUDs) are associated with increased risk of migraine headache.[40] In combination with low zinc levels, excess copper has been suggested as a precipitating factor in migraines.[41] The menstrual cycle and contraceptive pills have been linked with migraines and are associated with imbalances in mineral levels, including zinc deficiency.[42]

At high levels, zinc might enhance the toxicity of glutamate and other excitotoxins, so supplementation should not exceed 15–25 mg per day. This intake is below the NOAEL (no observed adverse effects level) and is generally considered safe. Migraineurs should avoid supplements containing zinc aspartate, which combines zinc with a known migraine trigger.

Coenzyme Q_{10}

Coenzyme Q_{10} (CoQ_{10}) supplements can prevent migraines. CoQ_{10} is a potent antioxidant used by mitochondria in the cells for energy production. When excitotoxins are applied to brain cells, the cells are unable to maintain their energy production. CoQ_{10} can help restore the cells' energy generation capability and prevent free-radical damage. Furthermore, a combination of CoQ_{10} and vitamin B_3 (niacin) maintains energy production and prevents nerve cell death.[43]

An "open label" study is one in which both doctor and patients know which medications are being given. In one such study, thirty-two patients had a frequency of two to eight migraine attacks each month.[44] They were supplemented with CoQ_{10} (150 mg each day) for three months, and 61 percent had their number of headache days per month reduced by more than half. The average number of attacks also dropped from 4.85 at baseline to 2.95 a month over the last two months of the study. This increase in effectiveness over time is not surprising, since CoQ_{10} is fat soluble and somewhat difficult to absorb, so it takes time to accumulate in the body.[45] Moreover, migraine preventative therapies often take weeks to achieve maximum effectiveness.

A randomized trial of CoQ_{10} in forty-three migraine patients also reported benefit. The existing attack frequency was 2–8 times a month. The trial compared CoQ_{10} (100 mg three times per day) with a placebo, and 48 percent of subjects reported having less than half as many attacks as before. In the third treatment month, CoQ_{10} was superior to the placebo for attack frequency, headache days, and days with nausea.[46] Another recent study also reported a positive effect for CoQ_{10} in preventing migraines.[47] CoQ_{10} levels were assessed in 1,550 children and young people (3–22 years old) with migraine. The normal range for CoQ_{10} plasma levels is 0.5–1.5 mg/L, but 74 percent of study patients had low or deficient levels. The patients with low CoQ_{10} levels were given supplements of 1–3 mg/kg/day and their average serum CoQ_{10} levels rose to 1.20 mg/L. Headache frequency and disability both showed a highly significant decrease, as the average number of headache days per month fell from nineteen to thirteen (about half of the supplement takers reported a 50 percent reduction in headaches).

Bandolier, an organization promoting evidence-based medicine, claimed the drug topiramate significantly reduced the frequency of migraine: about half of patients reported at least a 50 percent reduction in the frequency of attacks.[48] The results from the drug and the CoQ_{10} studies are similar. However, Bandolier, while accepting the drug's effects, described the CoQ_{10} results as providing a "smidgin" of evidence. There appears to be no rational justification for such a biased conclusion. It is worth noting that there are few reported side effects from CoQ_{10}, and none are serious, whereas topiramate's side effects include paraesthesia (pins and needles sensation), fatigue, dizziness, drowsiness, decreased appetite, weight loss, nausea, insomnia, depression, lack of concentration, memory difficulties, abdominal pain, nervousness, confusion, agitation, and visual and speech disturbances. Make your own judgment on migraine therapies—relying on medical authorities can be harmful to your health.

CoQ_{10} is relatively expensive and the intake required to prevent migraine could be anywhere between 150 mg and 1,200 mg a day. To assist absorption, take CoQ_{10} in divided doses, preferably with fish oil or a similar source of fat. CoQ_{10} is generally recognized as safe; it is non-hazardous and nontoxic.[49]

Riboflavin

Vitamin B_2 (riboflavin) is a water-soluble vitamin that can prevent migraine attacks. It is used in several energy and antioxidant pathways in cells.[50] Cells generate energy from the slow "burning" of food in oxidation-reduction reactions. The main process in these reactions is the transfer of electrons from one molecule to another. Riboflavin is involved in many of these essential reactions.[51] It is needed for the breakdown of fats, proteins, and sugars to generate energy. Riboflavin is a dietary antioxidant and is needed by the enzyme glutathione reductase, which is used to reduce the main intracellular antioxidant, glutathione. Not surprisingly, deficiency of glutathione can cause increased oxidative stress.[52] This vitamin also aids the liver in detoxifying drugs and removing poisons.

Riboflavin increases the mitochondrial energy reserve in the brain cells. As we have seen, changes in the brain's mitochondria and the loss of energy this produces may be involved in migraine. The oxygen metabolism of cortical brain cells changes during the aura and into a migraine attack. Since riboflavin is essential for the normal functioning of mitochondria, it is reasonable to suggest that supplementing with the vitamin might prevent migraine.

The B vitamins often work together and riboflavin deficiency affects many systems and interferes with the role of several other B vitamins. Riboflavin is involved in the biochemistry of vitamins B_3 (niacin), B_6 (pyridoxine), and folic acid. Adequate riboflavin is needed to lower blood levels of homocysteine[53], which is thought to be a factor in heart disease. Symptoms of vitamin B_2 deficiency include cracks and sores on the lips, tongue reddening and inflammation, and sore throat. The skin may be moist, scaly, and inflamed, and blood vessels may invade the cornea of the eye. The number of red blood cells may be reduced but the cell size is normal, as is the amount of oxygen-carrying hemoglobin.

People with migraines may have a higher need for this vitamin and an inadequate supply may increase their susceptibility to migraine attacks. Notably, deficiency of riboflavin may lower nitric oxide release and blood vessel dilation in migraine. Such changes are common to both preeclampsia and migraine. Pregnant women deficient in riboflavin are at increased risk of preeclampsia.[54] In this condition, blood pressure is raised, the hands and face swell, and protein is found in the urine. While blood pressure elevation is a defining symptom of the disease, it may be secondary to kidney and liver damage. Preeclampsia may progress to eclampsia, a life-threatening condition with increased risk of hemorrhage and seizures. In one study, supplementing with low doses (15 mg) of riboflavin reduced the incidence of preeclampsia, but the result was not considered significant.[55] A larger dose or riboflavin in a B-vitamin combination may have been more effective.

Vitamin B_2 supplements prevent migraine. Researchers studied fifty-four adults with repeated migraine attacks, giving riboflavin (400 mg per day) for three months in a randomized controlled trial.[56] The riboflavin outperformed the placebo, lowering the number of attacks and the number of headache days; 15 percent of the placebo subjects responded positively compared with 59 percent of those taking riboflavin. As expected from vitamin therapy, there were no major side effects, though three minor adverse events were noted. As with most preventative treatments, the maximum benefit seemed to be in the third month, suggesting that people should take riboflavin for several weeks to experience the full effect.

In 2004, a further study replicated the finding that riboflavin helps prevent migraine attacks.[57] In twenty-three patients, the average frequency of migraine attack was lower after supplementation with B_2 (400 mg per day) for three months. This was an open label study in which the subjects knew they were treated and there were no placebo controls. Riboflavin reduced the frequency, duration, and intensity of headaches. Headache frequency was lowered from four to two days per month. However, the intensity and duration of actual attacks did not differ significantly.

There is evidence that riboflavin can safely lower the frequency of migraine attacks. Experimental data suggests that this simple B

THE MACARENA APPROACH

When leading scientist Bruce Ames reported the results of a two-nutrient combination on aging rats, he said the results were astonishing: "With the two supplements together, these old rats got up and did the Macarena. The brain looks better, they are full of energy—everything we looked at looks more like a young animal." (For those who don't know, the Macarena is a lively, Latin-influenced line dance that was popular in the 1990s.) The two rejuvenating nutrients were alpha-lipoic acid and acetyl-L-carnitine.

Results from experiments suggesting that CoQ_{10} or riboflavin might correct mitochondrial energy problems in migraine are also relevant to these Macarena nutrients. Lipoic acid crosses the blood-brain barrier and acts as a powerful antioxidant in mitochondria, while acetyl-L-carnitine revs up the mitochondria, producing more energy, though at the expense of some oxidation. Fortunately, alpha-lipoic acid restricts or prevents the damage that could otherwise be caused by this induced oxidation. The combination allows damaged or aged mitochondria to function almost as well as those of healthy young animals. Consequently, there is an excellent theoretical case for the use of this combination in migraine.

A recent open study suggested that alpha-lipoic acid might be a useful migraine preventative.[58] Five centers studied fifty-four migraine patients (forty-three without aura and eleven with aura). Eighteen patients received a placebo and twenty-six were given alpha-lipoic acid (600 mg per day) for three months. A significant reduction in attack frequency, number of headache days, and severity was demonstrated in the alpha-lipoic acid group, whereas no change was noted in the placebo group. No adverse effects were reported. The authors concluded that alpha-lipoic acid may be beneficial in migraine prophylaxis and recommended further trials for confirmation.

Acetyl-L-carnitine is a form of activated carnitine, which is used by mitochondria for transporting fatty acids. The Headache Center at Cincinnati Children's Hospital carried out a study of carnitine in two girls with migraine.[59] The girls had experienced fatigue and muscle cramps in addition to side effects from their migraine drugs. Their carnitine levels were found to be low, so supplementation was used to correct the deficiency. Both showed a reduction in headache frequency and their symptoms improved. Carnitine supplementation has also been recommended for MELAS syndrome, a mitochondrial disorder with migraines as a symptom.[60] There have been no clinical studies combining the use of alpha-lipoic acid and acetyl-L-carnitine in migraine at this time. However, for some, the combination may turn out to be helpful.

vitamin could be as effective as many commonly used drugs, without the drugs' side effects. The maximum single dose of oral riboflavin likely to be absorbed is about 30 mg. However, by taking a riboflavin supplement with every meal, the amount absorbed will be far more and may yield greater benefits. For maximum anti-migraine effect, riboflavin should probably be taken in divided doses or in a slow-release formulation. The studies on single doses may underestimate riboflavin's anti-migraine action. Taking 30–50 mg of riboflavin, four or more times a day (total 120–200 mg per day), might provide the greatest benefit.

MELATONIN—THE DARK HORMONE

Melatonin, a hormone found in many animals and plants, may help prevent migraines. Melatonin is released by the pineal gland, a small structure at the base of the brain. It is important in regulating the sleep-wake cycle (the biological clock or main controller is in the brain). One of its main uses as a supplement is to counteract jetlag. Synthesis of melatonin in the pineal gland is related to sleep: it occurs during darkness and is inhibited by light—even low light levels can block melatonin production, as can exposure to electric lights. Blood melatonin levels are highest in the middle of the night and fall as daylight returns.

This hormone has several roles in the body; it is a widespread antioxidant, protecting the cells' DNA and mitochondria. These antioxidant and protective mechanisms are particularly relevant to the brain and may be important in migraine. One of the benefits of melatonin is that it can cross the blood-brain barrier and cell membranes. In some senses, melatonin is a pure antioxidant: when it is oxidized, it changes into a different molecule. The oxidation of melatonin produces other substances that may also act as antioxidants, a mechanism that generates a protective antioxidant cascade. This has the advantage that melatonin always acts as a protective antioxidant, and does not become a damaging oxidant. Melatonin can increase the life span of mice; whether it might produce similar life extension in humans is not known.

Its antioxidant properties alone suggest that melatonin would be likely to help migraine sufferers. An additional benefit is that melatonin may prevent glutamate toxicity.[61] Studies suggest it could be helpful for preventing migraine.[62] In part, melatonin supplements may prevent migraines by helping to stabilize the circadian sleep-wake cycles[63], as lack of sleep or too much sleep are both potent migraine triggers.

Low melatonin levels increase the risk of migraines. In one study, the nighttime melatonin levels of ninety-three migraine patients were found to be lower than those of normal controls.[64] Migraineurs who were depressed showed the greatest deficiency. In a second study, ten female migraine sufferers showed lower nighttime melatonin levels throughout the female cycle compared with controls.[65] Similar results showing decreased melatonin in migraineurs have been reported in other studies, along with suggestions that it is lowered further during a migraine attack.[66] The finding of low melatonin levels in migraine sufferers leads directly to the idea that supplementation may be beneficial. In a study of six female migraine patients and nine controls, melatonin infusions led to relief of symptoms in all six patients.[67]

Another study researched the effects of melatonin on headache in thirty patients, and reports from two patients are particularly interesting. A 54-year-old man suffered twice-weekly disabling migraine attacks without aura. With melatonin supplements, he reported only three migraine attacks in twelve months. A 60-year-old man had experienced cluster headaches since his forties. His episodes lasted about two months and occurred twice a year. After starting melatonin supplementation, just one cluster episode was reported, which lasted only five days.[68]

In children, melatonin has produced results comparable to those of the best preventative drugs. A recent study examined twenty-two headache sufferers, 6–16 years old. Thirteen of the children had recurrent migraines without aura, one child had migraine with aura, and the remaining children had chronic tension-type headache. They received melatonin (3 mg) each evening for three months. Fourteen of the children reported that their attacks were reduced by more than 50 percent, and four had no headaches during the trial.[69]

The dose of melatonin used to treat insomnia is quite low, perhaps 0.3 mg each night.[70] Available supplement doses are often higher, typically in the range of 1–10 mg. Use of high-dose melatonin to prevent migraine is generally considered safe. Individuals vary in their response to melatonin and it may be necessary to start with a low dose, perhaps 1 mg, and increase to the level that provides maximum relief without daytime drowsiness. It is reported that high doses of melatonin can bleed into the daytime, making the person feel drowsy or tired. An effective dose should produce restful sleep without daytime irritability or fatigue. However, the likelihood of daytime fatigue may be overstated, as other experiments report people taking up to 40 mg before sleep without any carryover fatigue.[71] Even exceedingly high doses can be well tolerated.[72] Importantly for migraine, the brain-protecting effects of melatonin are dose related.[73] Clearly, it should be taken shortly before retiring for sleep and should not be taken immediately before driving or operating dangerous machinery.

Melatonin shows promise as a migraine preventative agent. Unfortunately, once again, a full evaluation is not possible since clinical trials are lacking. The medical establishment has failed the population of migraine sufferers by not investigating fully another potentially effective and safe therapy.

HERBAL MEDICINE

Feverfew

Feverfew (*Tanacetum parthenium*) is a traditional, daisy-like herb with a long medical history of use as a treatment for headache, digestive upset, and arthritis. The way it works has not been established, but ideas include the standard explanations of changes in brain serotonin and lowering inflammation.[74] There are several bioactive substances in feverfew, including parthenolide and tanetin. Feverfew is not normally used to try to abort a migraine but for headache prevention. The active substances may take several weeks to become effective, however.

There is reasonable evidence for the efficacy of feverfew in preventing migraines, despite claims to the contrary by conventional medicine.[75] In a clinical trial lasting twenty-four weeks, seventeen patients took either freeze-dried feverfew leaves (100 mg) or a placebo each day.[76] The subjects had previously been regular feverfew users. The number of attacks increased significantly when subjects stopped taking feverfew and switched to a placebo; there was no change in the subjects who continued to take the herb. Five of eight subjects reported a good to excellent response with feverfew, and it seems likely that feverfew was preventing the headaches. An alternative possibility, that subjects taking the placebo suffered feverfew withdrawal symptoms, is not corroborated by other trials and anecdotal reports suggesting feverfew prevents migraines.

A trial of fifty-seven migraine patients started with a two-month period in which all the subjects received feverfew (100 mg) a day. The experimenters then evaluated the subjects' use of either feverfew or a placebo each day for two months.[77] After one month, the treatment groups were swapped. Feverfew resulted in a significant reduction in pain intensity compared to the placebo. Profound reductions in the severity of migraine symptoms were noted, including less vomiting, nausea, and sensitivity to noise and light. When the feverfew-treated patients transferred to the placebo, there was an increase in pain intensity and severity of the symptoms. Switching the placebo group to feverfew reduced their pain intensity and symptoms.

In another clinical trial, seventy-two patients used dried feverfew leaves or a placebo each day for eight months. Feverfew produced a highly significant reduction in headache frequency.[78] In a further study, an extract of feverfew was tested as a migraine preventative. After sixteen weeks, feverfew reduced the migraine frequency from 4.76 to 1.90 attacks per month.[79]

Feverfew is available in standardized extracts in 300–400 mg tablets to be taken once a day. If nutrients are not found to be effective in preventing migraine, herbal remedies such as feverfew can be considered a second line of defense, being safer than drugs. Feverfew should not be taken by pregnant women, as there is insufficient safety data.[80] It may cause the uterus to contract, increasing the risk of miscarriage or premature delivery.[81] No other serious side effects are expected with feverfew. Minor side effects include swelling and irritation of the mouth, with loss of taste, nausea, digestive problems, and bloating. Allergic reactions are also possible: I have experienced and seen feverfew cause pompholyx, a type of eczema, often affecting the hands or feet. While orthomolecular therapies have an excellent safety record, herbs may cause more problems. However, when compared with the number of major side effects from drugs, herbs are remarkably safe and often equally effective.

Butterbur

Butterbur (*Petasites hybridus*) belongs to the daisy family. Traditionally, Native Americans used butterbur as a treatment for inflammation and headache. Extracts of butterbur include petasin and isopetasin. Petasin may be a smooth muscle relaxant in addition to an anti-inflammatory agent. Butterbur root extracts are used as a treatment of migraine.[82]

A clinical trial of butterbur extract showed a reduction in the number of migraine attacks.[83] Sixty patients received either butterbur extract (two 25-mg tablets, twice daily) or a placebo for twelve weeks. The frequency of migraine attacks decreased by up to 60 percent compared to the baseline and no adverse events were reported. The analysis methods of the study were criticized, so an independent reanalysis was conducted, which found that the responder rate (at least a 50 percent reduction in migraine frequency) was 45 percent in the butterbur group and 15 percent in the placebo group.[84]

Another clinical trial compared different doses of butterbur extract (50 mg and 75 mg twice a day) with placebo in 245 migraineurs.[85] The age range was 18–65 years and the subjects had suffered a minimum of between two and six attacks in each of the preceding three months. Over four months, attack frequency was reduced by 48 percent for the 75-mg dose, 36 percent for the 50-mg dose, and 26 percent in the placebo group, an apparent dose-dependent effect. The proportion of patients who had their attack frequency cut in half after four months was 68 percent for those on the 75-mg dose. The results suggested a significant benefit of the 75-mg dose throughout the study.

The role of a butterbur root extract for migraine prevention has also been studied in children and adolescents.[86] The trial included 108 subjects, 6–17 years old, who had experienced severe migraines for at least a year. They were treated with 50–150 mg of butterbur root extract for four months. A reduction in migraine frequency of at least half occurred in 77 percent of the patients. After four months of treatment, 91 percent reported improvement.

For migraine prevention, 75 mg of butterbur extract each day appears to be more effective than lower doses. The most commonly reported side effect is burping.

NUTRIENTS, NOT DRUGS

Conventional medicine has produced minimal success for sufferers from migraine. Drug therapies provide only limited migraine prevention, and many nutrients appear to have equal preventive action at lower cost and with increased safety. Unfortunately, medical studies on nutrients in migraine prevention are sparse relative to the number of drug trials. Considering the disabling nature of the illness and its high frequency in the population, this lack of studies is indefensible. In this chapter, we have seen how a range of supplements may be useful in preventing migraine attacks. In many cases, clinical trials suggest that the effects are at least equal to those achieved with the most powerful drugs available, but with few, if any, side effects. Let us hope that in the near future physicians will acknowledge the limited progress with drugs and base their migraine therapy around nutrition.

CHAPTER 6

SUPPORTIVE NUTRITION

These small things—nutrition, place,
climate, recreation—are inconceivably
more important than everything one
has taken to be important so far.
—FRIEDRICH NIETZSCHE

A number of dietary supplements may be beneficial in the prevention or treatment of migraines. Furthermore, the underlying mechanisms of migraine may also point to potentially helpful supplements. One underlying mechanism is inflammation, so any anti-inflammatory supplement may be effective. Food substances can either encourage or inhibit inflammation—trans fats, for example, promote inflammation, whereas many spices are anti-inflammatory. Thus, a migraineur may benefit from a diet low in trans fats and high in anti-inflammatory foods and supplements. Other mechanisms of migraine involve brain neurotransmitters such as serotonin. Supplements, including 5-hydroxytryptophan (5-HTP), can increase serotonin levels in the brain (certain anti-migraine drugs target serotonin in this way) and could benefit migraineurs. And migraine is associated with severe pain, so supplements or herbs that relieve pain are obvious candidates for therapy.

In this chapter, we examine some of these substances to show how they may be of benefit in treating or preventing migraine headaches.

ABOLISH INFLAMMATION

Migraine is a disease of inflammation, so lowering the potential for inflammation is a primary approach to prevention and relief. Many nutritional supplements are predicted to be beneficial. Anti-inflammatory nutrients and herbs are common and have been tried in a variety of conditions, although there is a shortage of specific clinical studies on nutrition and migraine. Nevertheless, it is reasonable to suggest that anti-inflammatory supplements, such as turmeric, will provide substantial relief to migraineurs. There are physiological reasons why these supplements should work and, as the old saying goes, absence of evidence does not imply evidence of absence. While we wait the years necessary for these safe anti-inflammatory agents to be properly studied in migraines, people are free to experiment. Indeed, for a person wishing to obtain relief from migraine, self-experimentation is essential.

Anti-inflammatory drugs developed from the historical observation that certain plants could relieve pain, fever, and inflammation. The ancient Greeks, Sumerians, Assyrians, and Native Americans used extracts of willow bark for fever and pain. Willow bark contains salicylates, which were discovered and isolated in the middle of the nineteenth century, and from which aspirin (acetyl-salicylic acid) was developed. Aspirin led to the development of a large number of nonsteroidal anti-inflammatory drugs (NSAIDs).

In the 1970s, aspirin was found to inhibit the synthesis of prostaglandins, local hormones involved in inflammation. The discovery and isolation of prostaglandins simplified the search for new pain-killing drugs. Before then, new analgesics were found by screening, observation, or trial and error. The main limitation to the use of aspirin and related drugs was stomach upset and gastrointestinal side effects. Once prostaglandins were discovered, it became possible to design and target drugs more precisely. Scientists found that two main cyclo-oxygenase (COX) enzymes control the production of prostaglandins, COX-1 and COX-2. COX-1 maintains the stomach lining and regulates gut, vascular, and kidney functions; COX-2 promotes inflammation, pain, and fever.

The benefit from NSAIDs, such as aspirin or ibuprofen, comes from inhibiting COX-2 enzymes, thus preventing pain and inflammation. However, aspirin and most other NSAIDs also inhibit COX-1 enzymes, leading to stomach irritation and ulcers. Side effects of treating inflammatory diseases by blocking both COX-1 and COX-2 enzymes include kidney toxicity and peptic ulcers, in addition to stomach irritation and bleeding. Long-term use of these drugs to prevent migraines, or as a therapy for other chronic diseases, is therefore not appealing.

COX-1 inhibitors, such as NSAIDs, are effective against inflammation but have numerous and potentially serious side effects. Researchers therefore wondered whether developing drugs to preferentially block COX-2 might avoid the side effects of aspirin and other NSAIDs. They knew that this was possible, as turmeric extract (curcumin) has this ability.

By the year 2000, the introduction of selective COX-2 inhibitors appeared to have solved the problem. These drugs included Celebrex (celecoxib) and Vioxx (rofecoxib). They were claimed to block inflammation with fewer side effects and soon became popular with arthritis sufferers. The new drugs were commercial blockbusters, but cardiovascular side effects soon became apparent.[1] In 2004, Vioxx was withdrawn from the market because of serious side effects, including increased heart attack and stroke. Over five years, Vioxx was implicated in the deaths of about 100,000 people and in 160,000 heart attacks and strokes.[2]

Since the drug side effects became apparent, drug companies embarked on a search for safer options. The current search is for drugs that act on more than one inflammatory pathway, for example, COX and LOX (5-lipoxygenase), without the side effects of current medications. Drugs with this action are postulated to have a safe anti-inflammatory effect, be potentially curative in some rheumatic conditions, and protect the brain.[3]

In fact, such substances are already known to exist—they are safe, natural, low-cost nutritional supplements. The curry spice turmeric provides a natural alternative to these synthetic drugs and is thought to prevent heart disease, dementia, arthritis, and other degenerative diseases. However, it cannot be patented and hence there is no incentive for drug companies to fund its development, as an anti-migraine treatment. This contrast, between the effort expended to copy the action of nutrients and the failure to investigate fully the nutrients themselves, goes to the heart of the problems with current medical research.

Curcumin

Curcumin, a supplement derived from turmeric, holds great promise for the prevention and relief of migraine. Turmeric's characteristic yellow color comes from curcumin. The turmeric plant (*Curcuma longa*) is related to the ginger family and is found in India, where people have exploited it for around 5,000 years in cooking and as a paste to relieve inflammation and pain.[4] It is widely used as a household remedy and a headache treatment. In India, golden milk, flavored with turmeric paste, is taken for breakfast. Sweetened with honey, golden milk is also given to children who have suffered cuts or bruises, providing consolation and medication in one draught. For thousands of years, turmeric was believed to have health-giving properties and an ability to fight various diseases, including cancer and dementia.[5] It is used extensively in traditional Indian (Ayurvedic) medicine. Its applications include antiviral, antibacterial, and antiseptic treatments for cuts, burns, and bruises.[6] It is also used widely as a spice and dietary supplement.

Recent research into the properties of curcumin supports these ancient claims.[7] Curcumin has a powerful anti-inflammatory effect,[8] and researchers have demonstrated its efficacy in a number of diseases. In addition, curcumin is a powerful antioxidant. Research is under way to evaluate its benefits in dementia,[9] cancer,[10] and liver disorders.[11] Surprisingly, migraine does not seem to be a major concern or stimulus for research, despite the large number of anecdotal reports and turmeric's long history of use as a headache cure in Indian medicine.

Curcumin has not been subjected to clinical trials as a migraine treatment. Nevertheless, the actions of this supplement—including pain relief, brain protection, and inhibition of inflammation—all suggest it might help.

Curcumin's ability to relieve pain and reduce inflammation make it a likely candidate for preventing and alleviating migraine attacks. Curcumin readily crosses the blood-brain barrier and acts both as an antioxidant and as an anti-inflammatory agent.[12] Furthermore, it protects the brain from heavy metal poisoning[13] and from reductions in the blood supply.[14] Curcumin acts rather like a safe form of aspirin, but with more extensive anti-inflammatory actions. One effect of curcumin is to block the actions of the COX and LOX enzymes, similar to the aims of new anti-inflammatory drugs. Unlike the drugs, however, curcumin acts by affecting cellular controls rather than having a direct blocking effect on the receptor.[15]

Curcumin is exceptionally safe. There have been claims that, like most antioxidants, curcumin can act as an oxidant.[16] However, any assumption that such oxidant actions are harmful is overly simplistic: under certain circumstances, selective oxidation can be highly beneficial. It can destroy cancer cells, for example.[17] Curcumin's only reported toxicity involves mild nausea and diarrhea at high doses. At low intake levels, curcumin is advocated as a treatment for gastrointestinal problems.

Unfortunately, when taken orally, curcumin is not well absorbed from the gut.[18] For this reason, supplements sometimes contain a black pepper extract (piperine or bioperine), which can reportedly help increase absorption by up to twenty times.[19] However, piperine might also increase the absorption of certain prescribed drugs, such as phenytoin (an anti-epileptic) or propranolol (a beta-blocker used to control blood pressure).[20] For this reason, a physician should be consulted if piperine is to be taken alongside conventional drugs. A "new generation" curcumin supplement called BCM-95 may be well absorbed without piperine.[21] Another possible therapeutic approach would be to use liposomes to aid curcumin's absorption. Similarly, curcumin nanoparticles have been suggested for the treatment of cancer and other diseases.[22]

Since I was aware that curcumin could provide relief from severe back pain, I thought it might work against migraine. I therefore tried sublingual BCM-95 and found that it could abort a headache over a period of about two hours. If dissolved under the tongue, 400 mg of curcumin provided greater relief from a migraine attack than 30 mg of dihydrocodeine. However, the taste is relatively strong, as expected from a spice, and it leaves a yellow tongue; it might also stain false teeth, though I have no direct reports of this.

Curcumin is poorly absorbed and, to be effective, daily doses of perhaps 5 grams may be necessary for maximum relief. Lower intakes (1 gram or more) of BCM-95 or liposomal curcumin would be equally or more effective. Liposomal curcumin should increase the absorption at high intakes, without the effect of staining the tongue. A practical suggestion is to take curcumin supplements at the same time as a fish oil supplement, which may aid absorption and also help to lower inflammation. Curcumin is a highly promising, potential anti-migraine supplement that may be tried by anyone.

Fish Oil

As our grandmothers used to say, eating fish is good for the brain. Fish oil and other sources of omega-3 polyunsaturated fatty acids have beneficial effects on inflammation; they can also help relax blood vessels and prevent blood clotting.[23] Fish oils provide similar cardiovascular benefits to the much-hyped statin drugs. These properties make omega-3s potentially useful for preventing migraine.

Researchers studied the use of fish oil supplementation in twenty-seven adolescents who suffered from frequent migraines.[24] Two months of fish oil supplementation was followed by a washout period, and then by two months of olive oil, supposedly acting as a placebo. This is not an ideal procedure, since it is likely that the participants could tell the difference between the oils. Furthermore, olive oil may itself help prevent headaches, since it contains antioxidants and anti-inflammatory substances[25] and has properties similar to NSAIDs.[26] Compared with the adolescents' initial incidence of migraines, both the fish oil and the olive oil treatments reduced headache frequency. The reported improvement led the researchers to conclude that both fish oil and olive oil could be beneficial for recurrent migraines in adolescents.

In another study, patients were given either a 6-gram dose of omega-3 fatty acids or a placebo daily for sixteen weeks.[27] The total number of attacks during the four-month treatment period was significantly lower in the omega-3 group (5.95) than the placebo group

(7.05). Despite this positive result, the researchers claimed not to have confirmed the findings of previous studies based on the small number of patients. Strangely, the authors reported a statistically significant benefit, yet described their result as a "failure."

The available evidence suggests that migraineurs should supplement with fish oil, which appears to be effective in preventing headaches. Furthermore, supplementation provides additional health benefits. To be effective in lowering the incidence of migraine, up to about 6 grams of fish oil may be required each day. One suggestion is to use a combination of fish oil and magnesium taurate.[28] All three components of this combination (fish oil, magnesium, and the amino acid taurine) may help to damp down the neuronal hyperexcitability that precipitates migraine attacks. Since fish oil provides numerous other health benefits, it is worth trying as an approach to preventing migraine.

Boswellia

In the Christmas story, three wise men from the East, the Magi, brought presents of gold, frankincense, and myrrh to Bethlehem. The value of gold is obvious, but the purpose of the other items may be unclear in modern times. Myrrh was a highly valued reddish-brown resin made from the dried sap of the tree *Commiphora myrrha;* it was used at funerals as incense and for embalming bodies. The myrrh resin was also used for treating arthritis, bruises, aches and pains, and women's hormonal problems.

Frankincense is another resin, which comes from several species of *Boswellia,* a hardy, shrub-like tree that grows in demanding, rocky environments. Like myrrh, it is used in aromatherapy, but it is also available as boswellia herbal tablets. The symbolic use of frankincense in church services is interesting, as it has recently been found to be a psychoactive drug that can alleviate depression or anxiety. For centuries, boswellia has been used in folk medicine for chronic inflammation.

Since migraine is an inflammatory condition, boswellia is potentially beneficial to sufferers. Inflammation is a characteristic of many illnesses, so the potential medical applications of boswellia are increasing with time. Currently, they include Crohn's disease,[29] chronic colitis,[30] and cancer.[31] It is also reported to be helpful in arthritis, heart disease, and asthma.[32] In a placebo-controlled trial, seventy patients with arthritis of the knee showed improved pain scores and functioning with a derivative of boswellia called 5-Loxin (250 mg daily). Boswellia also appears to have a direct action on the brain, helping stabilize emotions.

Boswellia fights inflammation in a different way from NSAIDs: it inhibits the inflammatory enzyme 5-LOX. Extracts of boswellia are anti-inflammatory without being antioxidants and act on the inflammatory LOX pathway.[33] Boswellia also inhibits other inflammation-promoting enzymes known to be involved in chronic disease.

Currently, there are no trials of boswellia for migraines, even though its anti-inflammatory action suggests it would be beneficial. Despite this, it is currently being promoted as an anti-migraine treatment. I have tried both boswellia and its derivative supplement (5-Loxin) and found them to be well tolerated and reasonably effective for prevention and relief of migraine. Since boswellia has an excellent safety profile and may be effective, it could be considered for those whose migraine does not respond to other treatments. Combination supplements of boswellia with curcumin are available. Typical daily intakes are 1 gram of boswellia extract or 75–250 mg of 5-Loxin. The alternative to self-experimentation is to wait ten years or longer in the hope that clinical trials will be undertaken.

Glucosamine and Chondroitin

Commonly taken for arthritis, both glucosamine and chondroitin have anti-inflammatory properties and are sometimes recommended for migraines. There is little recent conventional research into their effectiveness, although there is some clinical evidence that they may be helpful in prevention. One observation followed the use of glucosamine as a treatment for osteoarthritis, when doctors in the Brampton Pain Clinic, in Ontario, Canada, made a serendipitous observation.[34] They noticed that when a patient took glucosamine for osteoarthritis, the patient stopped having migraines. As a result, they treated a further ten migraine patients who were unresponsive

PEPPERS FOR MIGRAINE RELIEF?

Capsaicin is the substance that makes chili peppers hot. It is an irritant to humans and other mammals (although birds seem to be immune), producing a burning sensation in the mouth, eyes, or skin. Capsaicin and similar substances called capsaicinoids are produced by chili peppers, probably as a protective mechanism to stop them from being consumed by fungi or eaten by animals. Capsaicin is used as a non-lethal weapon in pepper sprays, but too much capsaicin can be fatal. The irritant nature of capsaicin provides a high degree of safety from accidental overdose. However, it is surprisingly common for people to consume large amounts, resulting in vomiting, nausea, abdominal pain, and burning diarrhea.

Despite its fierce reputation, scientists are hoping to use capsaicin to develop new anti-inflammatory painkillers for use in conditions such as arthritis. Capsaicin has been used to treat cluster headache: it was applied via the nose as an analgesic with reported success.[36] The positive findings in the cluster headache study led to a trial of intranasal capsaicin in chronic migraines. Eight patients with chronic migraine were assigned to either a capsaicin or placebo group. The capsaicin group received 100 microliters of an emulsion, containing 300 micrograms of capsaicin. All the patients treated with capsaicin reported a 50–80 percent improvement in their migraine.

Putting pure capsaicin up your nose is not recommended! If you want to try this substance, nasal sprays containing capsaicin are available for migraine relief. One of these was discovered by accident by a self-defense instructor named Wayne Perry, who appeared regularly on TV.[37] His specialty was to take part in demonstrations illustrating the effect of pepper sprays in self-defense. However, he had a cluster headache just before such a demonstration. After the reporter pepper sprayed in his face, Perry found that his headache disappeared almost immediately. As a result, he developed an anti-headache pepper spray.

to standard treatments for prevention or aborting a headache, with daily oral glucosamine. After four to six weeks, patients noted a substantial reduction in headache frequency and intensity. Anecdotally, I have tried glucosamine as a migraine preventative, with a reasonable response in apparently lowering the frequency and intensity of headaches.

Like glucosamine, chondroitin is often recommended for arthritis. As long ago as the 1930s, however, chondroitin was thought to prevent migraines. In 1941, thirty patients were given four 600-mg capsules of chondroitin, three times a day, after meals.[35] The patients included sixteen cases with migraine and fourteen with headaches of undiagnosed origin. After treatment varying from six months to three years, 67 percent had been completely relieved of their symptoms. In a further 13 percent, chondroitin was reported to be partially effective, while 20 percent reported no benefit. Those patients that did not respond to the supplement were given drug treatment. Modern medicine seems to have forgotten this result and there are no recent clinical trials.

Glucosamine (1,500 mg each day) and chondroitin (1,200 mg each day) may be considered for those with migraines that fail to respond to treatment.

SEROTONIN ENHANCEMENT

The use of serotonin-boosting supplements relies on the theory that low brain levels of the neurotransmitter serotonin are a critical factor in migraines. This idea has led to the introduction of some reasonably effective anti-migraine drugs, such as the triptans. However, serotonin levels may be a side issue when it comes to understanding migraine.

For those who want to achieve higher serotonin levels, 5-hydroxytryptophan (5-HTP) supplements are often recommended for migraine prevention. 5-HTP is a naturally occurring orthomolecular precursor substance, which the body uses to synthesize serotonin. This supplement has been used clinically for over three decades and is taken widely as a natural antidepressant and appetite suppressant. It is given as an aid to sleep and a therapy for depression.[38] As well as

increasing brain serotonin, it can increase levels of two other neurotransmitters, dopamine and noradrenaline.

There is evidence that 5-HTP supplementation may help prevent migraines.[39] One study showed that natural 5-HTP levels might
be lower during attacks of migraine with aura.[40] In another study,
a comparison with the beta-blocker propranolol concluded that,
although both were effective against migraines, the drug had the
superior performance.[41] Despite this limitation, 5-HTP was reported to provide an alternative approach.

A comparison of 5-HTP with methysergide, a drug used for prevention of migraines, was conducted in 124 patients.[42] The drug
gave a reported improvement in 75 percent of the patients, while the
benefits of 5-HTP were comparable at 71 percent. 5-HTP reduced
the intensity and duration of attacks though not their number. Since
side effects were lower with 5-HTP, it was suggested that it could be
a treatment of choice in migraine therapy.

Other studies of migraine have obtained positive results with 5-
HTP. One trial, involving thirty-one patients with chronic primary
headache, compared 5-HTP with a placebo.[43] The patients had
migraines (sixteen patients), mixed headaches (six patients), psychogenic headaches (five patients), and muscle contraction headaches
(four patients). 5-HTP was reported as more effective than the placebo for lowering headache frequency and severity, but the result
was not statistically significant. In the second month of the study,
nearly half the patients showed at least a 50 percent average reduction in headache symptoms. Once again, the mild and transient side
effects of 5-HTP, compared to those of conventional drugs, suggest
that it could be a suitable approach to prevention.

Some warnings are appropriate: supplementation with 5-HTP
might interact with other drugs that also increase serotonin and its
effects, including antidepressants (such as Prozac) or monoamine
oxidase (MAO) inhibitors. It may also interact with the herb St.
John's wort, which is sometimes recommended for migraines. Substances that increase serotonin can cause the rare but potentially life-
threatening serotonin syndrome, in which increased serotonin in the
brain and spinal cord result in overstimulation. Signs of serotonin
syndrome include high blood pressure, raised temperature, flushing,

dizziness, and disorientation. Fortunately, 5-HTP has not been specifically implicated in serotonin syndrome in humans.[44]

Substances that increase brain serotonin are not necessarily benign. Some groups of people react differently to serotonin increase, particularly those with autism or Asperger's syndrome. People with these conditions may process serotonin differently, and the side effects of serotonin-enhancing substances may be magnified.[45] The role of serotonin may be modified in the teenage years, suggesting that the effects could differ markedly between children and adults.[46]

5-HTP may be used as an alternative to serotonin-boosting drugs. I have used it to prevent my migraines but found I did not like its side effects; however, many individuals report benefit and use 5-HTP regularly. Supplements of 5-HTP from 50 to 100 mg are typically suggested, taken two or three times a day.

ADDITIONAL SUPPORTIVE NUTRIENTS

Some nutrients can specifically help prevent migraine attacks and these form the first line of a nutritional therapy. Some work better in combination with others. For example, magnesium provides a defense against excitotoxins and its actions are enhanced by zinc. It is important to take a holistic approach, combining supplements that support each other. Here, in a quick run through of the main vitamins and nutrients, we evaluate their individual contributions. Mostly, these requirements can be achieved with a good-quality daily multivitamin and a B-complex supplement. However, there are exceptions; for example, vitamin C is needed in much higher amounts than found in multivitamins.

Vitamin A

There is little literature on the relationship between vitamin A and migraines. Vitamin A is generally safe but, being fat soluble, it does have the theoretical potential for overdose. Pregnant women need to be careful not to consume too much vitamin A, which can cause birth defects. For others, the available toxicity data show that the risks of overdose are almost infinitesimally small, and the dangers of vitamins are overstated and overplayed. However, reports suggest that overdosing on vitamin A can act as a migraine trigger in some people.[47] Conversely, deficiency of vitamin A can aggravate inflammation[48] and may therefore contribute to the frequency and severity of migraine attacks. Vitamin A is an essential part of the diet and, in general, deficiency is more to be feared than excess.

B Vitamins

The B-vitamin group contains several substances that may help prevent or treat migraines. Regular supplementation may have additional benefits in lowering the incidence of migraine attacks.

Thiamine—Thiamine (vitamin B_1) is a water-soluble B vitamin, one of the earliest to be discovered. Too little thiamine leads to beriberi, a disease that has been recorded for several thousand years. Beriberi is a neurological disease that also affects the gut and cardiovascular system. There are two forms:

- Dry beriberi causes peripheral neuropathy, with symptoms of burning feet, enhanced reflexes, and loss of sensation in the hands and feet. In severe cases, seizures may occur.

- When cardiovascular symptoms are more evident, it is called wet beriberi. Symptoms include congestive heart failure, heart enlargement, and increased heart rate.

Thiamine helps the body produce cellular energy from food and is essential for the functioning of several enzymes in mitochondria, the cell's power center. Despite the role of mitochondria in neural energy production, little direct research has been conducted on thiamine and migraines. Around 1950, there were studies claiming migraines had been treated successfully using vitamin B_1 and head traction manipulation, though no follow-up reports were published.[49] In a more recent study, twelve patients with mitochondrial disease were treated with supplements that included thiamine, riboflavin, coenzyme Q_{10}, vitamin C, and a high-fat diet.[50] Patients identified with a particular gene mutation (3243A>G) reported fewer migraine headaches with these supplements.

Riboflavin (Vitamin B_2)—Riboflavin is a water-soluble vitamin that can prevent migraine attacks. It was described in some detail in the chapter on prevention (see Chapter 5).

Pantothenic Acid (Vitamin B_5)—Pantothenic Acid is critical to cells, as it is needed to form coenzyme A, which is used to generate energy from food in mitochondria. This vitamin's role in metabolism and the generation of cellular energy may suggest a role in migraine prevention, similar to that of CoQ_{10}. Vitamin B_5 is also used for cellular communication, detoxifying drugs, and the synthesis of neurotransmitters, steroids, melatonin, and hemoglobin. Deficiency of B_5 is rare, as it is found in many foods, reflecting its necessity to life. In cases of severe, prolonged malnutrition, B_5 deficiency is associated with tiredness, headache, insomnia, and numbness of the extremities. Vitamin B_5 is formed by bacteria in the intestines and some may be also absorbed from this source. Pantothenic acid is safe in high doses and 1,200 mg a day is generally well tolerated, although such doses may cause heartburn and nausea. However, doses in excess of 10,000 mg (10 grams) may cause diarrhea.

Vitamin B_6—Vitamin B_6 is a water-soluble vitamin that comes in three main forms: pyridoxine, pyridoxal, and pyridoxamine. Neuropsychiatric disorders, including seizures, migraine, chronic pain, and depression, have been linked to B_6 deficiency.[51] In light of this, it has been used to reduce the incidence of epileptic attacks.[52] Importantly, vitamin B_6 is essential for the synthesis of niacin (vitamin B_3), which may be used to abort migraine headaches. (Niacin is described more fully in the following chapter.)

Vitamin B_6 is involved in the functioning of about 100 enzymes that are used in essential chemical reactions. It is needed to synthesize glucose, which is of particular relevance to those considering low-carbohydrate Atkins-style diets as a preventative approach to migraines or epilepsy. Such diets require broad-spectrum supplemental support, especially of vitamin C, magnesium, and antioxidants. B_6 is essential to cardiovascular health, particularly for avoiding increased homocysteine in the blood, a recently discovered risk factor for atherosclerosis, heart attack, and stroke.

Women are more prone to migraines than men, which may be

largely attributable to varying hormone levels during their monthly cycles. Many women take vitamin B_6 to lower the side effects of oral contraceptives and to treat premenstrual syndrome (PMS). In the latter half of the female cycle, women can experience depression, irritability, fatigue, and other symptoms. These symptoms typically end with the monthly period, but may also be associated with migraines. Clinical trials of B_6 show some evidence for benefit in reducing the effects of PMS.[53] Despite the close association between migraines and the female cycle, there appear to be no specific studies on B_6 and menstrual migraines.

Since vitamin B_6 is involved in the synthesis of serotonin and noradrenaline, it has been suggested that deficiency may be a factor in depression. However, clinical trials have not shown that B_6 supplementation is an effective treatment for depression, though it may be beneficial in hormone-related depression in women.[54] It could therefore be of some use to female migraineurs.

Serotonin is thought to be involved in the pathology of migraine, although its role may be secondary. The synthesis of other neurotransmitters, such as dopamine, noradrenaline, and GABA (gamma-aminobutyric acid), are also dependent on vitamin B_6. GABA is of particular interest, since, as the main inhibitory neurotransmitter, it helps balance glutamate (the excitatory amino acid implicated in migraines). Vitamin B_6 has a long history of use for treating morning sickness during pregnancy.[55] Since nausea and vomiting are defining symptoms of migraine, B_6 might be useful, although there are few, if any, specific studies in this area.

Generally, the B vitamins have low toxicity, since they are water soluble and are typically excreted rapidly. However, people taking large doses (greater than 500–1,000 mg a day) of vitamin B_6 for long periods can suffer from a temporary sensory neuropathy. This can lead to pain and numbness in the hands and feet and to difficulty in walking. In rare cases, people taking about 500 mg daily for months have developed the condition. There have been no validated reports of sensory neuropathy at doses up to 200 mg a day.[56]

Biotin—Biotin (vitamin B_7 or vitamin H) is occasionally included in anti-migraine treatments, although there appears to be no supporting evidence from clinical trials. Biotin is not known to be toxic and the lack of adverse effects means that there is no tolerable upper level of intake.[57]

Folic Acid—Folic acid (folate or vitamin B$_9$) may play a role in preventing migraine and its complications. Some people with migraine have specific gene types (alleles) associated with folic acid metabolism and with low levels of folic acid.[58] In addition, increasing intake of folic acid can lower the increased risk of stroke in migraine sufferers,[59] so adequate levels are vital. The use of folic acid to prevent migraines has been suggested, but, once again, clinical trials are awaited. A trial of folate in sixteen children with a genetic predisposition for migraine suggested a resolution or reduction in migraine attacks.[60] Until the results of clinical trials are available, migraineurs would be well advised to supplement with folic acid.

Vitamin C

Vitamin C is the main water-soluble antioxidant in the diet, and high intakes are beneficial to migraine sufferers. Frederick R. Klenner, M.D., one of the first doctors to use high doses of vitamin C in therapy, was a migraine sufferer. Massive doses of vitamin C can control many diseases and infections, but unfortunately this effect does not appear to apply with the same force to prevention or treatment of migraines. Nevertheless, gram-level intakes of vitamin C can provide protective antioxidant support and help overcome the stress of a migraine attack.

When I have a migraine and need to work, I take very large doses of vitamin C. But even large oral doses (10–20 grams) are not effective at aborting migraines. They do not remove the pain or other effects, though they can make the symptoms more bearable. Normal vitamin C tablets limit the dose that can be absorbed before bowel tolerance levels are reached, but liposomal formulations help increase absorption and sustain high blood levels. Taken in large doses, liposomal C appears to potentiate the effects of other treatments. Currently, most liposomal vitamin C contains sodium ascorbate, the sodium salt form. If liposomal magnesium ascorbate becomes available, this might provide a safe migraine abortive, as injected magnesium sulfate is an established way of stopping migraine attacks.

The limiting effect for oral doses is that vitamin C acts as a laxative. There is little evidence available to determine the optimal intake, but a healthy adult appears to need at least 3 grams a day, in divided doses, and the required intake increases with illness.[61] So, a person at higher-than-normal risk of heart disease or infection could beneficially consume more than 10 grams of vitamin C a day.[62] Government recommendations on vitamin C and other nutrients are based on misleading experiments, performed over a decade ago and urgently need updating.[63]

Vitamin D

Vitamin D helps regulate the body's calcium and phosphate levels and is important for maintaining strong bones and teeth. It is formed by the action of sunlight on the skin. Because it is fat soluble, any excess is stored in the body, so it does not need to be taken every day. Despite this, perhaps partly because people avoid the sun for fear of getting skin cancer, vitamin D deficiency has been described as a modern pandemic, causing disease and illness. The claim that people should avoid sunlight to prevent melanoma and other skin cancers is greatly overstated. Vitamin D helps prevent cancer and this effect generally outweighs the risk of reasonable exposure to sunlight. Studies suggest that lack of vitamin D contributes to many of the world's chronic debilitating diseases, including rickets in children and bone weakness and fractures in adults. Deficiency has also been linked to increased risk of common cancers, autoimmune diseases, high blood pressure, and infectious diseases, such as influenza.[64]

Vitamin D may help prevent migraines. In one study, two post-menopausal women were described as developing frequent and excruciating migraine headaches.[65] The first was stricken following hormone replacement therapy with estrogen, the second after a stroke. Both women were treated with vitamin D and calcium, which provided a dramatic reduction in headache frequency and duration. The relief achieved was most likely due to the vitamin D. Magnesium, rather than calcium, is associated with migraine relief, while calcium competes with magnesium for absorption and is involved directly in the pathology of migraines. Vitamin D, on the other hand, affects magnesium absorption, which may help lower the incidence of migraines.[66]

Most people do not obtain sufficient vitamin D from food and the government recommendations for daily intake of vitamin D are inadequate. The two main forms of vitamin D are D_2 (ergocalciferol) and D_3 (cholecalciferol). Vitamin D_3 is the most effective form and can be obtained by exposure to the sun's ultraviolet (UVB) radiation or from supplements. Since exposure to excessive sun can age the skin or may be limited in many areas of the world, supplementation is important. On balance, vitamin D may be helpful for migraineurs, either directly or by increasing magnesium levels.

Vitamin E

Vitamin E may play a key role in keeping migraineurs healthy. Vitamin E and a form of CoQ_{10} prevent the toxic effects of excitotoxins, such as glutamate, on nerve cells.[67] Vitamin E may additionally support the actions of CoQ_{10} by acting as a lipid-soluble antioxidant. These antioxidants enter the brain, and clinical data on migraine and their ability to protect brain cells is overdue.

Vitamin E does not exist as a single element in the diet. Rather, it is the name given to a number of dietary components that prevent oxidation of fat in the body. The designation "vitamin E" is typically used to cover a group of four dietary substances called tocopherols (alpha-, beta-, gamma-, and delta-tocopherol). However, there is a second variant group called tocotrienols (alpha-, beta-, gamma-, and delta-tocotrienol), each of which is also "vitamin E." These substances (and many synthetic variants) each have unique vitamin E activity.

Conventional medicine tends to ignore the various forms of vitamin E, concentrating only on alpha-tocopherol. Apparently, the justification for this is that alpha-tocopherol is more actively retained in the body. This means that claims that vitamin E is ineffective in preventing heart disease and other diseases are generally invalid, because such claims typically apply only to synthetic alpha-tocopherol. As a result, the potential benefits of vitamin E have been obscured for decades. Thus, while vitamin E is often recommended as a supplement for migraines, there is little direct clinical data.

Vitamin K

Vitamin K is fat-soluble vitamin that gets its name from *koagula-tion,* the German spelling of "coagulation." This vitamin is essential for normal blood clotting and seems to be involved in migraines. Although some authors have claimed that vitamin K intake should be limited[68], there is little supporting evidence for this. Increased clumping of red blood cells may be a factor in migraine, but vitamin K does not cause such abnormal clotting. Moreover, it is an essential factor in the diet.

Warfarin is a vitamin K antagonist best known as rat poison: when used for rodent control, it blocks the rats' blood-clotting mechanism, causing them to bleed to death. In humans, low doses are used to prevent strokes, although intake has to be monitored carefully or the patient would suffer the same fate as the unfortunate rats. There are clinical reports of migraine frequency being reduced when people are on warfarin.[69] One study of three patients with cluster headache reported that two were headache free on warfarin, while the third experienced an initial increase in frequency followed by a long remission.[70] As explained earlier, cluster headache is a sporadic illness, occurring in clusters, with long periods of remission. It may be that the reports of benefit in cluster headache are describing the natural end of a period of headaches rather than a direct effect of the medication. The drug is claimed to have abolished migraines in one patient,[71] and anticoagulant therapy appears to have lowered the number of attacks.[72] Anticoagulants have also been proposed as a therapy for preventing migraines.[73] However, the anticoagulant drug approach carries the risk of bleeding complications and cannot be recommended.

A study of 574 Italians, ages fifty-five and older, including 111 people with a history of migraines, found that migraineurs face an enhanced risk of developing small clots in their veins (venous thromboembolism).[74] Small blood clots could potentially cause interruption or restriction of blood and oxygen to the brain and may cause local release of glutamate, oxidation damage, and inflammation, leading to a migraine attack. One model of migraine is that it is caused by abnormal blood clotting. However, it is unclear whether such clotting is a precipitating factor or a result of the inflammation and stress arising from the illness.

Inhibition of abnormal clotting can be more safely and effectively achieved with suitable nutrients, including CoQ_{10}, fish oil, ginger, garlic, *Ginkgo biloba*, green tea extract, magnesium, vitamins C and E, and so on. Many of these supplements are recommended for migraine relief.

TAURINE AND MIGRAINES

Taurine is a common dietary amino acid that has been proposed to have anti-migraine and anti-epileptic effects. In particular, it may dampen neuronal hyperexcitation, helping to reduce the effects of spreading depression associated with migraines.[75] The magnesium salt of taurine, magnesium taurate, taken in combination with fish oils, has been suggested as a migraine preventative.[76]

Researchers have found that taurine, glycine, and glutamine levels are increased in migraine patients.[77] Severe migraine is associated with lower levels of taurine in the brain than milder attacks.[78] Higher levels of brain taurine may inhibit the attack. Migraine patients excrete less taurine in their urine than healthy people do.

Since there is limited information about taurine in migraine, it is useful to look at its role in the related brain excitatory disease epilepsy. Taurine prevents seizures in mice given kainic acid, a glutamate-like excitotoxin.[79] Taurine acts on one of the major inhibitory receptors in the brain and can prevent the epileptic activity induced by lowering magnesium levels in brain tissues.[80] Injected taurine was found to prevent epilepsy in mice, whereas taurine given in drinking water over a four-week period failed to decrease the number of seizures.[81] In human epileptics, short-term positive results have been reported for taurine, but results have been less satisfactory in longer studies.[82] This is suggestive of a beneficial role for taurine in migraines, but once again medical research has failed to investigate it.

ANTIOXIDANTS

People with migraines may be particularly susceptible to oxidative stress. In order to test this idea, researchers performed a study to investigate an antioxidant formulation as a migraine preventative.[83] Their twelve patients had a long history of migraines, which were unresponsive to multiple conventional treatments. For three months, the subjects were treated with ten antioxidant capsules per day, each containing pine bark extract (120 mg), vitamin C (60 mg), and vitamin E (30 IU). The subjects continued their existing drug therapy. Over the treatment period, the patients showed significant improvements, with reductions in the number of headache days and the severity of attacks.

Ginkgo biloba leaves provide an herbal antioxidant that has long been used for vascular and neurological conditions. Anecdotal reports suggest that ginkgo prevents migraine, and it is widely used for this property.[84] However, a side effect of ginkgo is headache. There appear to be no conventional clinical trials.

Many of the substances that are used for migraine prevention or aborting an attack have antioxidant properties. This is clear for nutritional supplements such as CoQ_{10}, but can also apply to drugs (sumatriptan, the well-known migraine-aborting drug, is an antioxidant). The role of antioxidants in migraine therapy is largely unexplored.

HORMONE THERAPY?

Forms of herbal-based hormone replacement or modification are sometimes used for migraine prevention, particularly for menstrual migraines. Such substances include soy isoflavones, dong quai, and black cohosh. Dehydroepiandrosterone (DHEA) is a precursor to male and female sex hormones, and DHEA supplements have been used as an anti-migraine therapy. Similarly, conventional hormone replacement is sometimes prescribed for menopausal migraines. Clinical trials suggest that these natural hormone therapies provide effectiveness similar to other preventative therapies.[85]

One of the few beneficial aspects of migraine is that it is associated with a reduction of breast cancer in women. This 30 percent risk reduction appears to be connected to lower levels of estrogen and progesterone.[86]

Hormone therapies are more suitable for women than men and may be contraindicated in those with a propensity to breast cancer. The caution here is consistent with concerns about the long-term effects of additional hormones. However, hormones can be effective and may be recommended by doctors and health-care professionals. Individuals will need to decide whether the possible anti-migraine benefits of hormone replacement might be outweighed by the potentially increased cancer risk.

COMBINING THERAPIES

One of the themes of this book is that combination therapies can be effective against migraines. One beneficial combination of a vitamin, a mineral, and an herb is commonly used to prevent migraines—a "triple therapy" consisting of riboflavin (vitamin B_2), magnesium, and feverfew. The triple therapy combination has been studied in clinical trials. In one study, a daily dose of riboflavin (400 mg), magnesium (300 mg), and feverfew (100 mg) was tested for the ability to prevent migraine. However, a dose of riboflavin alone showed comparable benefits to the combination.[87]

A combination of feverfew and white willow (which is related to aspirin) was described as showing "remarkable efficacy" in preventing migraines. In an open-label trial, twelve migraine patients were given feverfew (300 mg) and white willow (300 mg) twice daily.[88] In nine patients, the frequency of attack was significantly reduced, by 57.2 percent after six weeks and by 61.7 percent after twelve weeks. A reduction in frequency of at least half was reported in 70 percent of the subjects. Migraine intensity was also reduced significantly in all patients, as was the duration of attacks. Patients tolerated the treatment well with no adverse events.

Combining nutritional therapies can mean that the benefits of the different supplements are additive. This synergy is most likely to occur when the way in which each supplement works differs. For example, curcumin's main action is to prevent inflammation, magnesium inhibits the NMDA (N-methyl D-aspartate) receptor, and CoQ_{10} is a mitochondrial antioxidant. Combining supplements with such different mechanisms of action is likely to provide effective migraine prevention. However, for maximum utility, they need to be taken for a period of perhaps three months, so there is often no "quick fix" for a migraineur.

When drugs are combined, interactions between them can generate side effects. By contrast, most nutrients can be combined without fear of even minor side effects. They are, after all, nutrients needed by the body for its normal functions. High-dose intakes of some nutrients do pose health issues, but these can be checked with a physician or other health-care provider. Herbal approaches are intermediate in terms of safety: herbs are not inherently safe, and just because something is natural, it does not mean it is harmless. However, herbs are generally safer than drugs and often have a long history of use.

CHAPTER 7

STOPPING AN ATTACK

Pharmaceutical companies are very annoyed
with niacin because their products
have to compete with it.
—ABRAM HOFFER, M.D., PH.D.

If used in the early stages of a migraine attack, dietary supplements can often stop it in its tracks. Unfortunately, once an attack has become established, such attempts are far less effective. One reason for this is that absorption of oral medications is blocked during an attack, for example, oral analgesics, and often fail to stop a migraine. This could be because the body misinterprets migraine symptoms as poisoning, so it shuts down the stomach as a protective measure. Vomiting, another common symptom of migraines, removes potential toxins from the body. However, drugs may be ejected similarly. One way around this problem is to use injected treatments—injected magnesium sulfate is an effective migraine abortive, at least the equal of comparable anti-migraine drugs. Another solution is to drink a cup of coffee, which might help absorption of analgesics as well as having limited anti-migraine effects.

The migraineur may face several forms of prejudice from the medical profession. The first is their inability to accept the disabling and painful nature of the illness. Second, there is an unwillingness to accept that available evidence suggests sufferers can gain at least the same level of benefit from nutrition and supplements as from drugs. The medical establishment has failed to investigate nutritional and related treatments for migraines, even though it is one of the most frequently disabling conditions.

In the last chapter, it was related that curcumin, when taken sublingually or possibly in liposomal form, can abort a migraine attack. Several grams of BCM-95 curcumin taken orally can also abort an attack if it is absorbed. In this chapter, some additional nutritionally based approaches are described. For purposes of comparison with natural remedies, we begin with a brief description of some notable drugs and their drawbacks. It is worth noting that in many cases, anti-migraine drugs can cause medication overuse headaches, which occur every day. Others result in rebound headaches, in which the migraine attack is initially aborted, only to return the following day. Natural nutritional therapies provide a safe and effective alternative.

CONVENTIONAL DRUGS AND THEIR DRAWBACKS

Triptans

Triptans (sumatriptan, zolmitriptan, and naratriptan) represent a major advance in conventional drug treatment for migraines. These drugs constrict arteries in the brain and can stop the pain of a migraine. Triptans increase brain serotonin and constrict blood vessels, limiting the flow of oxygen and other nutrients. Importantly, this constriction is not limited to blood vessels in the head—coronary blood vessels supplying the heart are also narrowed, which prevents the use of these drugs in people at risk of heart attack.[1] Constriction of vessels in the esophagus and lungs has also been noted, and there have been reports of chest pain and heart anomalies.[2]

At the time triptans were introduced, the prevailing model for migraine was that changes in brain serotonin led to dilation of blood vessels. Triptans affect a particular type of serotonin receptor that was thought to be involved. Earlier drugs used in migraine, such as the ergot derivatives, also act on serotonin receptors and constrict blood vessels. Typically, however, drugs have multiple actions and the triptans are no exception. It now seems that triptans abort migraines by inhibiting signals from the trigeminal nerve, which may be because triptans block the release of a local hormone involved in inflammation (calcitonin gene-related peptide or CGRP). The benefits of these drugs may thus be fortuitous and unrelated to the conventional explanation.

Triptans can abort a migraine attack, but the headache often returns within six hours to two days. These rebound migraines are common and occur in 20 to 50 percent of patients. Taking an additional dose for the second rebound migraine can be effective. However, the second dose may simply delay the process, leading to an additional rebound migraine.[3] I have found that the relief they provide is neutralized by side effects, including reduced clarity of thinking and some less-than-pleasant psychogenic effects. These drugs have recognized side effects (drowsiness, weakness, dizziness, flushing, heart rate alterations) and can produce strange, unwelcome feelings as they relieve the attack. Triptans are far more expensive than nonsteroidal anti-inflammatory drugs (NSAIDs), which may be used to treat an acute migraine attack with similar effectiveness. Triptans should not be used to prevent attacks as overuse can cause severe medical complications.

Analgesics

Many people with headache find relief with simple painkillers, such as aspirin, ibuprofen, and paracetamol (acetaminophen). In many cases, over-the-counter analgesics also contain caffeine, which may provide greater relief than the painkillers. However, turmeric (curcumin) and other nutrients can be safer and more effective at relieving pain and inflammation than aspirin and ibuprofen.

These drugs are usually effective in tension headaches. Similarly, physiotherapy may help where frequent or chronic tension-type headache is associated with muscle or joint problems. Changes in lifestyle, relaxation, and cognitive therapy can provide stress-coping strategies and prevent these headaches. However, tension headaches are not migraines, which are often far less responsive to relaxation.

Analgesics are typically of limited help with migraines. During a migraine attack, absorption from the gut can be compromised and the painkiller will prove ineffective as it stays in the stomach until the attack is resolved. In addition, holding aspirin or other NSAIDs in the stomach for long periods can cause erosion of the stomach wall, leading to ulcers. One medical approach to avoid this and aid absorption (slightly) is to use soluble formulations. In some cases, when oral symptomatic relief is not possible, anti-inflammatory drugs may be given by rectal suppository.[4]

There is an additional problem with paracetamol, a commonly used painkiller. As explained earlier, paracetamol is highly toxic and even small overdoses can lead to liver damage. During a migraine attack, a person could easily lose track of the number of tablets taken and might accidentally overdose. While suffering an attack, a migraineur may be tempted to take a higher dose in the hope of gaining some additional relief. Furthermore, all the tablets taken during the course of the attack, over many hours, can stay in the stomach, increasing the risk of overdose. A high dose of drugs could be released into the body as the attack subsides.

This danger could be avoided if manufacturers added a paracetamol antidote to the tablets; the food supplement L-methionine, for example. The antidote is inexpensive and effective, but drug companies generally do not include it in their formulations. Other supplements that act as paracetamol antidotes are N-acetyl-cysteine (NAC), alpha-lipoic acid, and vitamin C. People using paracetamol regularly should consider taking such supplements to help protect them from drug side effects. Clearly, migraine sufferers should also be careful not to take more than the recommended dose of paracetamol.

Antiemetic Drugs

Antiemetics are substances that prevent nausea and vomiting. Physicians sometimes prescribe antiemetics, such as metoclopramide or domperidone, to prevent nausea and sickness in migraines and other conditions. Unfortunately, these drugs have numerous side effects. Considering just metoclopramide, major side effects include dystonia (slow, twisting muscle movements), increased levels of prolactin (a hormone associated with lactation), neuroleptic malignant syndrome (muscle rigidity, fever, delirium), depression, lowered mental alertness, movement and muscle tension disorders, and high blood pressure.

A person suffering nausea with migraine has good reason to prefer a natural alternative, such as the spice ginger, to such anti-nausea medications.

NATURAL MIGRAINE REMEDIES

Ginger

Ginger (*Zingiber officinale*) is used in cooking, eaten as a delicacy, and has a long history as a medicine. It is also an effective antiemetic: it is the treatment most commonly recommended for nausea and vomiting by health food stores and is a widely used therapy for migraine.[5] There are several good reasons to consider using ginger. Migraines typically involve nausea, vomiting, and dizziness, and ginger is a traditional herbal remedy for morning sickness, motion sickness, and vomiting.[6] Migraine is an inflammatory illness and ginger is an anti-inflammatory agent, which, like aspirin and the other NSAIDs, inhibits both COX-1 and COX-2 enzymes.[7] Furthermore, the processes leading to a migraine attack involve oxidation and ginger has antioxidant properties.[8]

While your family physician may suggest ginger as a possible treatment, medical science has largely ignored this spice. A search of the National Library of Medicine for papers on the use of ginger in migraine produced only a handful. The oldest paper, from 1990, suggested ginger might be both a preventative therapy and an abortant for migraine attacks, without negative side effects.[9] Another was a general paper on the potential for herbs to interact with drugs[10], while a third was critical of health food store recommendations in migraine and pregnancy.[11] Conventional medicine apparently has little interest in evaluating this commonly used therapy, despite migraine being a widespread and debilitating illness.

In addition to being free from side effects, ginger has a pleasant taste and can be used routinely. Tablets of concentrated ginger are available from heath food stores, and these can be taken early in an attack or as a preventative measure. A drink of sliced ginger root in hot water is an agreeable way of taking ginger. Ginger is generally safe, but excessive intake should be avoided by people on warfarin or those with gallstones.

Niacin

Niacin (vitamin B_3) is a water-soluble vitamin that comes in several forms, including niacin (nicotinic acid) and nicotinamide. Despite the name and chemical similarity, the effect of nicotinamide is not related to nicotine, the drug found in tobacco. The body uses niacin to form two important molecules, called nicotinamide adenine dinucleotide (NAD) and nicotinamide adenine dinucleotide phosphate (NADP). These chemicals are essential for energy production in the cell and for the production of antioxidants. NAD is often found in energy-producing reactions involving the oxidation of food. The NADP form is involved in antioxidant reactions and those that synthesize large molecules. Niacin can be synthesized in the liver from the amino acid tryptophan, which is found in dietary protein. Synthesis of niacin depends on the availability of vitamins B_2 and B_6 and, indirectly, of iron.

Niacin is an excellent supplement for fending off a migraine attack—taken at an early stage, niacin can abort a migraine. Jonathan Prousky, BPHE, M.Sc., N.D., of the Canadian College of Naturopathic Medicine, has investigated this approach to migraine relief. Dr. Prousky found that, if taken early, niacin can abort migraine attacks. However, large doses of niacin cause skin flushing, which can be extremely disconcerting. The skin becomes very hot and red, and may itch slightly. This is a harmless reaction and experienced users might even enjoy it. However, people taking a high dose for the first time have occasionally been sufficiently alarmed to attend an emergency room. Almost one in five people taking a large dose of niacin for the first time found the flushing intolerable and would not try it again.[12] For migraineurs, the niacin flush can be most welcome.

Niacin's anti-migraine effect seems to be related to its flushing action. One explanation for the action of niacin is that the skin flushing is caused by a mild inflammation, which may release anti-inflammatory substances into the bloodstream. Niacin may affect CGRP activity in the trigeminal nerve, a factor in inflammation and pain. The resultant anti-inflammatory response may damp down the migraine. In addition, the nerve may receive additional blood flow and oxygenation from the dilated blood vessels.

While niacin has not been generally considered as a migraine preventative by the mainstream medical community, it is often used by migraineurs, who claim benefits. In 2003, the Mayo Clinic reported a dramatic response to slow-release niacin. Researchers suggested that this response to niacin is noteworthy, as preventative medication has not made the same level of improvement as migraine-aborting drugs.[13] The case study concerned a 62-year-old woman who had suffered migraine headaches for almost forty years. She approached the Mayo Clinic for help with her increasingly frequent attacks. The woman had not used standard preventative medicine, but had taken triptans for relief of acute attacks. At first, she suffered one to two headaches each month, which lasted one to two days and came with standard migraine symptoms of "nausea, vomiting, photophobia, phonophobia, and exacerbation with movement." She had no clear headache triggers.

Nine months before visiting the Mayo Clinic, the woman's migraine attacks had become more frequent but less severe. She experienced a headache two or three times each week, which was not alleviated by sumatriptan and ice packs, though zolmitriptan did help. The change in her illness followed two stressful life events: the death of a relative and moving back home. By chance, a friend of hers was taking niacin to lower cholesterol and he mentioned that the niacin cleared up his migraines. As a result, she tried slow-release niacin (375 mg twice daily) and, amazingly, after forty years of suffering, her migraines stopped. Two weeks later, she visited the Mayo Clinic, who advised her to continue with her regimen of 750 mg per day. However, she decided to lower the dose to 375 mg a day, because by then she had been headache free for a month. Over the next two months, she had two mild migraines, which were resolved with zolmitriptan. Since then, she continued taking sustained-release niacin and reported being headache free and having no adverse effects.

Such is the lack of investigation of nutritional therapies that the Mayo Clinic researchers could find only one reference to niacin used alone as a treatment for migraines.[14] They described this report as "anecdotal," which is a term used in medical jargon to suggest unreliable evidence. They also claimed to have found only a single reference to the use of niacin as a supportive treatment for migraine.[15] However, a Google search on niacin and migraine, undertaken for this book, produced three-quarters of a million pages. There are, in fact, numerous early reports of people who have used niacin to prevent or relieve migraines. A 2005 literature review found fourteen articles on niacin in migraine and headache.[16]

In 1944, an early study was conducted on niacin and migraines.[17] Based on medical records and subjective assessment of twenty-one patients, 81 percent reported a positive response to niacin. In 1946, injections of niacin (100 mg) were tried in 100 patients with headache and 75 percent of the treated individuals reported complete relief.[18] There were few side effects and the benefits of the niacin appeared to be linked with the associated skin flush. In 1949, a study of fifteen patients suggested niacin is beneficial in the treatment of migraines.[19] Thirteen patients (87 percent) reported benefits, and twenty-seven out of thirty-one migraines were relieved. In 1951, a study suggested that niacin was beneficial in tension headaches.[20] Of twenty-two subjects receiving 100–200 mg of niacin, 59 percent reported a positive response. Moreover, 77 percent said their headaches were relieved by niacin. Similar studies of niacin for emotional or tension-type headaches and depression followed; these also suggested positive benefits.[21]

In 1991, a researcher who suffered migraines reported that 300–500 mg of niacin, allowed to dissolve in the mouth, resolved the headache.[22] Absorption through the tissues of the mouth is an effective method of taking nutrients, often more effective than just swallowing the tablet. In this case, by avoiding delayed absorption through the gut, niacin may be more effective at aborting a migraine attack. Sucking or chewing a niacin tablet may facilitate its uptake and could be effective even when stomach absorption is compromised. In 2003, Dr. Prousky reported two patients who aborted migraines using 500 mg oral doses of niacin, taken during the early stages.[23]

People need about 10 mg of niacin each day to prevent acute deficiency disease (pellagra). However, healthy young adults need up to 16 mg a day to provide consistent metabolism of this vitamin.[24] Some scientists think that these levels are too low and suggest that biochemical indicators (levels of NAD and NADP) could indicate that higher intakes are needed. However, as with other estimates of daily requirements, which are based on acute disease or simple biochemical measures, such low intakes of niacin may result in chronic disease (such as schizophrenia and other psychoses).

Niacin taken at the start of a migraine attack may provide complete relief. People with migraines may require more niacin than the government recommended upper limit. Those unused to niacin supplements should try low doses of around 50–100 mg, to help acclimatize them to the surprising effects of the niacin flush. Even with these low doses, the flush can be somewhat dramatic in sensitive individuals. Having induced a flush with a low dose, higher doses can be used to prevent or abort a migraine attack. Twice daily supplements of 500 mg may help prevent headaches. Niacin doses of 500–1,000 mg can be used to induce a flush at the start of a migraine attack. The dose may be repeated at half hourly intervals if a flush does not occur.

Niacin Safety

A high oral dose of niacin (100–1,000 mg) will produce an immediate flushing of the skin in most people. This flushing is somewhat variable: higher doses may be needed on some days to achieve the same level of flush. For the migraineur, flushing with niacin is not a side effect but an aim, as it is necessary to gain the associated relief of migraine. Remember, it is important that people be introduced to niacin tentatively, with low initial doses, in order to become accustomed to milder flushing effects before taking higher doses. There are forms of vitamin B_3 described as "no-flush niacin," but these may be ineffective.

Minor side effects to niacin have been noted, including dry skin, skin rashes, short episodes of lowered blood pressure, and reduced glucose tolerance. Diabetics considering use of high-dose niacin should note that it might cause decreased insulin sensitivity. High-dose niacin may be contraindicated in gout, as it may increase uric acid levels. There are reports of some degree of liver damage and jaundice at high intakes (750 mg or more daily) of niacin, if sustained for months.[25] People with liver disease should avoid large doses of niacin supplements unless they are suggested by their physician. Slow-release tablets may be of greater concern, but reports of severe hepatitis are for much larger doses (3–6 grams) taken for long periods (months or years).[26] Other side effects include nausea and vomiting. Standard niacin tablets are used at higher doses and are believed to be safer. However, the side effects may have been overstated, as orthomolecular pioneer Abram Hoffer, M.D., Ph.D., who treated patients with high-dose niacin for many years, reported that he had not seen a single case of liver toxicity. Compared with typical anti-migraine drugs, niacin is a very safe molecule.

Vitamin B$_{12}$

Vitamin B$_{12}$, also known as cobalamin, may be effective for prevention and acute treatment of migraines. In particular, it may modify the effects of nitric oxide (NO), preventing the inflammation that is characteristic of migraine. Nitric oxide is a small gaseous molecule that promotes inflammation, expands local blood vessels, and can cause headache. The explosive nitroglycerin induces a form of migraine by releasing NO, a fact that throws some light on the mechanisms underlying migraines.

Long ago, people working in nitroglycerin manufacturing plants discovered that this substance can cause headaches. Since the 1870s, nitroglycerin has been used as a drug, to dilate blood vessels in the heart and other tissues; under its alternative name of glyceryl trinitrate, it is still used to treat angina. If people who normally suffer from migraine with aura are given glyceryl trinitrate, a migraine without aura is produced.[27] This suggests that NO initiates inflammation rather than cortical spreading depression. People who suffer from migraines are sensitive to the action of NO, leading to the suggestion that the release of nitric oxide may be responsible for migraine pain.[28] Fortunately, vitamin B$_{12}$ may modify the effects of nitric oxide, and prevent the inflammation that is characteristic of migraine.

Several studies of B_{12} and headache from the 1950s are listed in medical libraries[29], but they have not been followed up by substantial recent research. In one recent trial, the effect of intranasal vitamin B_{12} was studied in twenty migraine patients.[30] The patients had histories of between two and eight migraine attacks each month. After three months of supplementation with B_{12} (1 mg per day), the frequency of migraines in 53 percent of patients was reduced by more than half; 63 percent had a reduction in attack frequency of more than 30 percent. The duration of migraine attacks, number of migraine days, and number of medication doses used for acute treatment each month were also reduced.

Vitamin B_{12} deficiency is common: more than one person in ten over the age of sixty is deficient. One reason for the widespread deficiency is that B_{12} is poorly absorbed from the gut. Pernicious anemia (a lack of red blood cells), which results from B_{12} deficiency, occurs in about 2 percent of people over the age of sixty. The risk of pernicious anemia runs in families, which suggests a genetic component for deficiency. Vitamin B_{12} deficiency also affects the brain and nervous system, causing numbness, tingling of the arms and legs, and difficulty walking. Over a period of years, it can also produce loss of memory and dementia. Restoring B_{12} might not reverse these changes, which suggests that permanent brain damage might occur. These nervous system changes can occur without other symptoms of deficiency. Depression is a symptom of both migraines and B_{12} deficiency. Three in ten women hospitalized for depression had low levels of B_{12} and deficiency can greatly increase the risk of depression.[31]

Vitamin B_{12} cannot be synthesized by humans, though it is produced by bacteria. Unlike many water-soluble vitamins, however, vitamin B_{12} is stored in the body, and this can be sufficient to prevent deficiency over years of inadequate intake. This vitamin is found in fish, meat, and milk, but is low or absent in most vegetables. Vegans, in particular, may need supplements. Since absorption of vitamin B_{12} from food is lowered as we age, people over the age of fifty might also benefit from supplementation.

The U.S. government does not set an upper limit for intake of vitamin B_{12}. Standard treatment of pernicious anemia involves injections of B_{12}, but oral supplementation is a viable alternative (about 1 percent of a large oral dose will be absorbed). In treatment of deficiency, doses of 1 mg (1,000 micrograms) or more are given daily. Alternatively, doses of 1 mg are given each month by intramuscular injection. In healthy people, large intakes have not been associated with adverse effects.

Vitamin B_{12} is a relatively large and complex molecule that contains cobalt. It comes in several forms, including cyanocobalamin and methylcobalamin. In supplements, cyanocobalamin is the most common form and this is converted to the active form, methylcobalamin, in the body. Vitamin B_{12} should be considered as a treatment option for migraine sufferers. I often take 5 mg of B_{12} sublingually (by placing the tablet under my tongue) if I feel a migraine coming on. It does not abort the headache but can reduce its symptoms. Migraineurs may be short of vitamin B_{12} and could benefit from supplementation.

While the available clinical data on vitamin B_{12} and migraine is limited, there is sound support for its mechanism of action. There is little risk of side effects and the potential for a lowering of migraine-associated disability.

Feverfew and Ginger

Although feverfew and ginger are not normally considered as migraine abortives, a combination of the two may be effective. In a recent study, thirty patients took ginger and feverfew sublingually during the early stages of a migraine. The authors reported that the blend was effective in aborting headaches.[32] About half the subjects were pain free after two hours, with one-third of the patients reporting only a mild headache. The combination is available as an over-the-counter medication.

This and other anecdotal reports from users of ginger suggest it may be an effective therapy. I have found ginger useful in preventing attacks and have used it in the early stages as an abortive medication. However, it is not possible to list the results of clinical trials, as they do not appear to have been performed.

Magnesium

Infusions of magnesium sulfate have been shown to stop migraine attacks.[33] However, it may not be easy to access this treatment via a conventional physician. Recently, I wanted to try injections of magnesium sulfate to abort my migraines. Although I know several ecological doctors in the United Kingdom who offer this treatment, I was interested to know whether I could get it on the National Health Service (the government health plan). Making an appointment with my family doctor, I saw a locum (temporary stand-in) instead of my usual general practitioner. I asked for a referral to a neurologist to avoid asking the doctor for a treatment of which he may have been unaware.

The neurologist I saw worked at a hospital where I had previously done research into aging and incontinence. The neurologist refused to speak to me until he had read the letter of introduction from the locum. When he had finished, the neurologist turned to me and said that he had never heard of magnesium being used as a migraine abortive, but had looked into its use and thought that it should work. I replied, "Of course it should, or I wouldn't be asking for it!" He added that he did not know why it wasn't standard therapy, but suggested that "presumably there's no money in it, or it hurts like hell." I noted that the profit motive was more likely.

Regrettably, there was a condition to letting me try magnesium injections: the neurologist demanded that I first try several conventional drugs, and only go on to the magnesium injections if the drugs proved ineffective. I said that this would be acceptable, provided the drugs' side effects were within reasonable bounds, to which he responded by pulling a face. I took this to mean that the drugs would have a long list of adverse effects. In fact, the first drug had headache as a side effect! The other main problems included paraesthesia (skin tingling), fatigue, dizziness, drowsiness, decreased appetite, weight loss, nausea, insomnia, depression, lack of concentration, memory difficulties, abdominal pain, nervousness, visual disturbances, speech disturbances, shaky movements, and weakness. (It is interesting that many of the side effects are symptoms of migraines.) The drug concerned was topiramate, an anti-epileptic medication described previously. Importantly, the drugs suggested to me as an alternative to magnesium were not for aborting a migraine attack, but for prevention.

Returning to my local doctor, I met with a different locum physician. This one suggested that there might be hidden side effects with magnesium that had not yet been discovered. (He was serious, and made this suggestion with a straight face.) This process is of concern because people with migraines often suffer a lack of interest or ignorance from the medical profession. Physicians can hide behind their years of medical training, which should make them more generally knowledgeable than the patient. However, in today's information age, the patient could have more specific information than the physician has. In my case, I can reasonably claim to have a degree of knowledge in this area.

Finding the conventional physicians' responses unacceptable, I decided to contact an ecological physician. Unfortunately, I found that this particular doctor was being subjected to a General Medical Council (GMC) hearing, accused of providing unconventional treatments, such as magnesium sulfate for migraine. I therefore organized a letter to the GMC, co-signed by several academic colleagues. We wrote to support the scientific basis of the doctor's treatments and offered to provide evidence; I don't know to what extent our letter was helpful, however, the case against the doctor was dropped. This example illustrates the difficulties of obtaining treatments that are not part of mainstream medical practice.

Research suggests that infusion of magnesium sulfate can bring about a rapid and sustained relief of an acute migraine or other headache.[34] In one placebo-controlled study, fifteen patients were given infusions of magnesium sulfate for treatment of acute migraine; all the patients in the treatment group responded.[35] The pain resolved completely in thirteen patients and was lowered in two patients. The accompanying symptoms disappeared in all of the patients. Unsurprisingly, patients with a migraine headache and low blood levels of free magnesium are more likely to respond to an intravenous infusion.[36] In one study, forty patients with acute migraine were given infusions of 1,000 milligrams of magnesium sulfate. Within fifteen minutes of the infusion, thirty-five patients reported a reduction in pain by half or more. The degree of benefit depended on the patients' blood magnesium levels as magnesium-deficient patients had a greater response.

An infusion of 1,000 mg of magnesium sulfate will abort a migraine attack in most patients. Such injections are suitable for acute treatment of a severe attack, rather than for prevention. (Oral magnesium supplements are more appropriate for migraine prevention.) Reduction of pain by 50 percent is reported to occur within fifteen minutes of the injection and complete or partial pain relief persists for up to twenty-four hours or more. There is some individual variation in response, depending on the condition of the individual—those with low blood magnesium levels will have a more pronounced response.

Doctors may be reluctant to provide this treatment because, while effective, it may be outside their normal scope of practice. There are some issues about delivering the injection, but as with diabetics and insulin, this is not necessarily restrictive. The slightly invasive nature of magnesium injections means that they need to be conducted under the supervision of a doctor. For those in North America whose family doctor is unwilling to provide the therapy, the treatment is available from orthomolecular practitioners. Those in Europe can consult the British Society for Ecological Medicine, who provide a list of practitioners. Such is the bias against nutritional therapies that patients may need to actively search to find a physician with suitable experience.

NUTRIENTS CAN STOP A MIGRAINE ATTACK

In addition to helping prevent migraines, nutrients can often be used to stop migraine attacks. Niacin, ginger and feverfew, and vitamin B_{12} may each be helpful. As we have seen, the evidence for magnesium injections compares well with corresponding drug therapy. Early clinical reports for niacin also seem to show a strong effect, but have not been followed up by clinical medicine. Similarly, sublingual B_{12} may be helpful but, once again, has been largely ignored clinically. As indicated earlier, liposomal curcumin or a large dose of the turmeric derivative BCM-95 may abort an attack (see Chapter 6).

Similarly, liposomal magnesium, when available, should provide a readily obtainable oral migraine abortive. There is also supporting evidence for the combined use of ginger and feverfew taken sublingually. Thus, when prevention of migraine breaks down, sufferers have several supplement options that might abort their headache.

CHAPTER 8

PHYSICAL THERAPIES FOR MIGRAINES

Do not undervalue the headache.
While it is at its sharpest it seems a bad investment;
but when relief begins, the unexpired remainder
is worth four dollars a minute.
—MARK TWAIN (1835–1910)

Migraine is a disease that touches all aspects of a person's life. It is affected by a large range of triggers, from duration of sleep to a change in the weather. The weather can bring on migraines when it is too cold, too hot, too sunny, or simply starting to rain. This sensitivity to physical changes in the environment suggests an approach to treatment. Physical change can be employed as therapy.

Migraine is such a difficult disease to prevent or to treat that it is necessary to use all appropriate means for therapy. While conventional medicine has a number of drugs that provide limited help, these may be considered secondary to therapeutic changes in nutrition and environment. This book is mainly concerned with how nutrition can be safely employed to prevent and treat migraines. However, we may extend this approach and combine nutrition with physical therapies, which provide an additional way for migraine sufferers to help themselves.

HYPOTHERMIA

While studying for my doctorate, I used to travel to medical school

131

on a motorcycle in all kinds of weather. Occasionally, I would set off on the thirty-mile ride home in subzero temperatures with a migraine. My choice was to either travel slowly and prolong the experience or ride quickly and suffer the wind chill. Mostly, I decided a shorter period was preferable. Ice would adhere to the outside of the helmet and to my moustache, and a pain-inducing blast of ice-cold air ran up my nose and around my head. However, the experience had one redeeming feature—it was an almost certain method of clearing a migraine.

A seventy-mile-per-hour motorcycle ride in subzero temperatures provides a rather extreme cooling of the head. It is unlikely to be taken up as a mainstream therapy for migraine, however. Despite this, it provided one of the most rapid ways of relieving a migraine I have ever experienced. I have tried a less extreme cooling by holding my head under a cold shower, which can produce an initial increase in the pain, not to mention increased blood pressure and a form of mild shock. Nevertheless, when the pain of the cooling subsides, there can be reasonable relief from the migraine.

Cryotherapy (the therapeutic use of cold) applied to the head has been studied as a method of relieving headaches. Ice packs are one of the most common non-drug methods for temporary relief of headache.[1] Most migraineurs have probably tried an ice pack, or perhaps a bag of frozen peas, for headache relief. An ice pack can be applied to a particular section of the head for relief, providing a gentler cooling than putting your head under a cold shower. To avoid getting frostbite, it is important that the ice does not come into direct contact with the skin: a protective layer of cloth should be used for this purpose. People with poor peripheral or skin circulation, such as diabetics, should not apply ice packs or similar cooling devices to their skin.

There are a number of positive reports of the benefits of head cooling in migraine.[2] In one short report by Peter Baxter, M.D., FRCPCH, and colleagues, three apparently normal children had headache on exercising.[3] The children were advised to try cooling their heads by pouring cold water over the head, immersing their heads in cold water, using an icepack, or applying a cold wet towel, when they felt a headache coming on. This was described as rapidly effective with no major side effects. One 12-year-old boy with exertion headaches had gained no benefit from drugs, including high-dose paracetamol, propranolol, and ibuprofen. Pizotifen and sumatriptan provided only transient help. Cooling the head was rapidly effective. Notably, the boy's father had used a cap dipped in cold water to relieve his headaches. A second 12-year-old boy's exertion headache had a similar lack of response to drug treatment and large benefit from wearing a cap dipped in cold water. This was confirmed by a 13-year-old who obtained some relief from painkillers but a substantial benefit from head cooling. The authors concluded, "For all types of headache, alternative or complementary modes of treatment may be effective but lack scientific evidence."

In another study, the use of cold wraps was studied in forty-five patients suffering from either migraines or migraines combined with chronic daily headache.[4] Although just 9 percent thought the cold wrap was completely effective, 55.5 percent found it moderately or mildly effective; 35.5 percent judged it ineffective. These results compare well with many conventional drug treatments.

A trial at the Diamond Headache Clinic, in Chicago, tested cold as a therapy for acute headache.[5] Ninety outpatients were spilt into three groups according to headache type: migraine, cluster, and mixed. Their normal medication was used alone for two attacks and in combination with application of a reusable, frozen gel pack for two attacks. The cool pack was reported to be effective by sixty-four patients; forty-seven reported an immediate decrease in pain; and fifty-seven patients described an overall decrease in pain. Cooling relieved all three headache types equally. Most patients (71 percent) said they would use a gel pack in future attacks.

There are various devices to cool a migraineur's head. One involves a vibrating curved pillow with a cooling or heating insert. However, vibrating one's head during a migraine attack is unlikely to be welcomed. Another is a pillow that places an ice pack at the back of the head, but this seems to cool a less than optimal part of the head for migraine relief. Cooling is generally most effective when applied to the front and top of the head. Based on a device tested in twenty-eight headache patients, which had a cooling compartment that encircled the head and part of the neck, with a separate warming compartment applied to the crown of the head.[6] Twenty patients had migraine, seven had tension headache, and one had cluster headache. This cooling/warming device reportedly provided relief in fifteen migraine patients, six tension headache patients, and the single cluster headache patient.

An interesting story concerns a Welsh builder, Hywel Edwards, who was diagnosed with migraine as a child. Throughout his upbringing, migraines disrupted his education. Later, loss of employment days and social events limited his enjoyment of life. Over time, Edwards tried many forms of pain and migraine relief with limited success. Experience suggested that cooling his head helped, but he found that most available methods were not practical, so Edwards decided to find a solution for himself.

Over three years of experimentation, he developed cooling caps that covered the main areas of the head, consisting of packets of cooling gel mounted in a Lycra helmet. The elasticity of the helmet allowed adjustment to the shape and size of his head, and it held the gel packs gently on its surface. Placing the prototype in the freezer, he awaited a migraine attack. When an attack came, he immediately tried his cap and could not believe the relief he experienced. The result was that he started his own small company to manufacture and supply caps to other migraine sufferers (MigraCap, Electronic Healing, www.electronichealing.org).

I have tried two types of Edwards' cooling caps and found them helpful. One covers the eyes and is useful for migraines with pain around the eyes or sinuses. The second allows the user to see normally and can be used when it is necessary to continue to be active. The cap that allows vision provides improved placement of the cooling pads along the path of the trigeminal nerve. These caps are convenient and cover the more important parts of the head, providing relief without drugs. Also, a cap is a one-time cost, whereas painkillers are a repeated expense. The caps can, of course, be used alongside nutritional approaches to aborting a migraine.

The main drawback of head-coolers is that they warm up over time. Depending on the ambient temperature, they cool the head for perhaps half an hour as they gradually go from ice cold to moderately cool. The intense cooling when taken straight from the freezer can cause an increased (cold) stimulus to the trigeminal nerve and may increase head pain initially, but it provides maximal benefit. Having two caps might be helpful, making it possible to use one while the other is in the freezer. Edwards' caps were useful and practical, and there are other ice gel packs, masks, or wraps, which serve a similar purpose. Migraineurs may want to consider why the medical profession and health-care industries have failed to provide such a simple, convenient approach.

PRESSURE

Pressure on the scalp has been used to relieve migraines, based on the idea that tension in the scalp muscles may contribute to headaches. In a study of twenty-five patients, researchers secured elastic bands around patients' heads with Velcro.[7] Firm rubber discs under the band applied local pressure over the area of maximum pain. Two patients dropped out of the trial because the band produced local discomfort. The twenty-three remaining patients used the band in three headaches each and their pain was checked over a period of half an hour. Of the sixty-nine headaches, sixty (87 percent) improved; nine showed no benefit. Of those people who had relief, 67 percent had reduced pain rated at over 80 percent improvement. The pain gradually increased when the tension in the band was released. Once again, these reported benefits compare well with conventional drug-based approaches.

TRANSCRANIAL MAGNETIC STIMULATION

Transcranial magnetic stimulation (TMS) may be able to stop the cortical spreading depression associated with migraines and relieve, or even prevent, migraine headaches. At the first symptom of a migraine, a hairdryer-sized device is placed on the head, administering brief, painless pulses of magnetic energy. TMS uses external magnets to induce weak electric currents in the brain, which excite the nerve cells. Rapidly changing magnetic fields create the electrical stimulation in the same way a dynamo generates an electrical current. A single pulse of TMS can excite brain cells in an area of the cortex. However, the effect of a single pulse is short lived, lasting about as long as the stimulation. For migraine therapy, repetitive transcranial magnetic stimulation (rTMS) is more appropriate and may be helpful in a range of neurological and related conditions. When pulses are repeated, they can produce either stimulation or long-term inhibition of brain cells. At high frequencies, stimulation with rTMS activates the underlying cortex, but at low frequencies the cortex is inhibited.[8]

Induced responses in the brain using electrical currents have been recognized for over a century, but medical interest began in about 1985. By that time, magnetic resonance imaging (MRI) was becoming established as a diagnostic tool and thus magnetic stimulation was considered more conventional. TMS has been used to show that migraineur brains are more easily excited than those of normal controls.[9] Stimulating the visual cortex with TMS produces apparent flashes of light called phosphenes. Migraineurs experience these flashes of light at lower TMS intensities than normal individuals.[10] Not all of the brain appears to be over-excitable in migraines—the visual cortex is more excitable than the area used for controlling movement, for example.[11] The source of this excitability is unclear. It could be that the brain cells are more excitable; alternatively, an inhibition mechanism could be absent.[12] A local shortage of magnesium, for example, would lower the inhibition, leading to greater excitability.

Repetitive transcranial magnetic stimulation may help prevent migraines. In a study of the effects of rTMS on depression, two patients suffered almost daily headaches.[13] When receiving rTMS, the patients' headache pain was significantly reduced, but returned to baseline when the treatment stopped. Later, when the patients were receiving rTMS about twice a week for depression, they experienced a sustained relief from their headaches. Another study of TMS indicated a strong reduction in pain.[14] The study involved forty-two patients with migraines. In the treatment group, pain decreased by 75 percent and TMS produced immediate and sustained reductions in migraine pain.

A study reported at the American Headache Society provided similar support for the use of TMS in migraines. Fifty migraine attacks were treated (twenty-one with placebo using a sham device and twenty-nine with TMS). Two hours after treatment, 69 percent of treated patients suffering migraine with aura reported that they were pain free or experienced only mild pain.[15] Patients also recorded improved symptoms such as a reduction in nausea. Although this sounds encouraging, it is worth pointing out that almost half of patients (48 percent) who used the placebo device, which looked similar but did not function, also reported benefit.

The electrical current produced by TMS carries a slight risk of causing seizures in susceptible individuals, a risk that is higher with rTMS, which is given at high intensity and frequency. Tension headaches, ringing in the ears, memory problems, and other cognitive effects have also been reported, though rarely, as side effects of rTMS. There are few long-term effects, but this may reflect limited experience with the technology. Applying radio waves and electrical signals to the head is becoming increasingly common with the use of cell phones and related devices. The worldwide safety implications of these new technologies are potentially enormous,[16] but the migraineur may consider such risks acceptable if the technology provides relief. The reported results, however, do not suggest a magic bullet but rather an approach that yields a typical treatment response. TMS is probably another therapy that may be effective in a proportion of migraine sufferers. Its advantage is that it is independent of drug-based treatments.

OXYGEN THERAPY

We all need oxygen to survive but, surprisingly, too much can be dangerous. High concentrations cause blood vessels in the brain to constrict, which is presumably a mechanism to protect brain tissues from overexposure. Since migraine involves dilation of blood vessels, it has been suggested that oxygen might be used as a treatment. Oxygen could also stimulate increased metabolism in brain cells. Oxygen therapy has several advantages as a potential migraine treatment but, for maximum benefit, it may need to be delivered at above atmospheric pressure.[17]

In 1981, work at the California Medical Clinic for Headache suggested that oxygen might be helpful for patients suffering with cluster headaches.[18] At the start of an attack, fifty-two patients were given access to masks delivering pure oxygen at a rate of seven liters per minute for fifteen minutes. The patients self-treated ten attacks and recorded how long it took their pain to subside. Three-quarters of the patients found substantial relief. By way of comparison, a second group of fifty patients treated their headaches with either a drug (sublingual ergotamine tartrate, every five minutes until headache subsided, maximum three tablets) or oxygen. In this trial, the patients reported slightly better results (82 percent obtained relief) for oxygen than for the drug (70 percent obtained relief). Although the oxygen was slightly more effective and had the advantage of fewer side effects, the authors suggested that the drug was more convenient.

More recently, researchers compared the use of high-pressure (hyperbaric) oxygen with that of oxygen at normal pressure (normobaric), because high pressure provides a greater level of blood oxygenation.[19] In a hyperbaric chamber, ten patients breathed pure oxygen at normal pressure, and ten breathed oxygen at twice atmospheric pressure.[20] Only one of the normal pressure group reported significant relief from headache, while nine of the hyperbaric group found relief. After the initial tests, the nine control patients who still had headaches were given hyperbaric oxygen and all reported improvement. The authors concluded that high-pressure oxygen might be useful for the abortive management of migraines.

Another study concerned the use of hyperbaric oxygen for prevention of migraines.[21] The authors reported a small, though statistically insignificant, reduction in the number of migraines after three sessions in a hyperbaric chamber. They concluded that their protocol of hyperbaric oxygen was not useful for migraine prevention.

According to these papers, high-pressure oxygen may be useful for treatment, though not prevention, of migraines, and normal-pressure oxygen may help cluster headaches. It is worth remembering that high-pressure oxygen is not without its dangers; for example, it can cause explosions. I have tried oxygen at normal pressure during migraines and found it ineffective. However, other migraineurs report that it provides useful relief.

ACUPUNCTURE

Acupuncture involves inserting and manipulating needles in specific points on the skin. It is used for treating numerous conditions, particularly (in the West) for relieving pain or inflammation. In traditional Chinese medicine, acupuncture points are positioned along meridians that channel *qi,* the "vital energy." Modern medicine has a problem with acupuncture, as the meridian lines do not appear to exist in the anatomy or tissues. For this reason, the ancient explanation does not make sense to conventional physicians and, despite its widespread use, acupuncture is considered controversial and denigrated by "skeptics." However, even those highly critical of alternative medicine are reluctantly admitting that it may be effective in some conditions.[22]

Lack of knowledge of the mechanism of action is a limitation, but understanding is not essential for acupuncture to be effective. One suggestion is that acupuncture can cause the release of endorphins, the body's natural opiates. Drugs such as heroin and morphine also act on endorphin receptors. Naloxone, a drug used to counteract the effects of opiate overdoses, blocks the action of morphine-like drugs. Interestingly, if naloxone is given to a patient who is having pain relieved by acupuncture, it can block the relief, resulting in increased pain.[23]

Acupuncture needles may stimulate local pain fibers, which feed back to the spinal cord and brain. These small signals may inhibit the larger pain signals from the headache.[24] Notably, the inhibition is suggested to occur in the brain stem, near to the site proposed by some as the origin of migraine. This idea follows from the gate control theory of pain—that the perception of pain can be turned off by the inhibitory effect of other signals.[25] An oft-quoted example occurs in professional sports where an injury may not cause pain until the end of the game. This mechanism provides an explanation for the pain insensitivity induced by meditation, drugs, or acupuncture, and might also explain why acupuncture's pain relief can be reversed by naloxone.

An alternate mechanism, also blocked by naloxone, would be central inhibition of pain in the brain. Brain imaging methods indicate that acupuncture acts on the brain[26] and there is also a suggestion that the effect varies with the acupuncture point stimulated.[27] In experiments with monkeys, acupuncture altered the response of neurons to painful stimuli[28], which suggests a direct physiological effect. Opiate-like endorphins are the most likely candidate for an induced chemical response, so the blocking of acupuncture's benefits with naloxone would be expected.

A 2006 study of acupuncture in migraines illustrates some of the difficulties of clinical investigation.[29] The aim was to compare the efficacy of two forms of acupuncture with that of standard treatments (beta-blockers, calcium channel blockers, or anti-epileptic drugs). The two forms of acupuncture were partly standardized traditional ("verum") acupuncture and partly standardized sham acupuncture. Patients with between two and six migraine attacks a month were randomly assigned to traditional acupuncture (313 patients), sham acupuncture (339 patients), or standard therapy (308 patients). The subjects received ten acupuncture treatments over six weeks or continuous drug therapy. Twenty-six weeks after starting treatment, there was an average reduction of 2.3 migraine days in the traditional acupuncture group, 1.5 days in the sham acupuncture group, and 2.1 days in the drug therapy group. The number of patients responding (with at least a 50 percent reduction of migraine days) was 47 percent in the traditional acupuncture group, 39 percent in the sham acupuncture group, and 40 percent in the drug therapy group. There was no statistical difference between the groups but all treatments were highly significantly effective. These results can be interpreted as showing that acupuncture is at least as effective as standard drug therapy, which is no better than placebo. These results may be somewhat depressing, but they should be kept in mind the next time someone suggests that conventional medicine has a more effective approach to preventing migraine than complementary medicine.

Acupuncture seems to be effective for prevention of nausea and vomiting, and thus may be of benefit in alleviating these symptoms of migraine. Stimulating an acupuncture point in the wrist has been studied for preventing delayed nausea and vomiting induced by cancer chemotherapy with positive results.[30] Reviews also suggest that acupuncture is equivalent to antiemetic drug therapy for preventing nausea and vomiting in chemotherapy, and, with training, acupuncture can be self-administered.[31]

While acupuncture's benefits on nausea are of interest, it is more often used by migraineurs to lower the frequency of attacks. A review of twenty-two trials of acupuncture in migraine suggested that patients benefited.[32] Notably, trials where acupuncture was compared to a standard drug treatment reported greater improvement and fewer side effects with acupuncture. One suggestion was that the correct placement of needles was less relevant in migraine therapy than is usually suggested by acupuncturists. Another review suggests that acupuncture is of benefit for headaches of unknown cause.[33]

Acupuncture provides a potential benefit to migraine sufferers. The effect may rival or even outshine the typical drugs used to prevent attacks. However, it would not be expected to work in all patients. When properly employed, its main attraction is like that of nutrient supplements: it provides a possible therapy with few, if any, side effects.

PHYSICAL THERAPIES PROVIDE RELIEF

Many physical therapies may provide relief from migraine and can be used in addition to vitamins and nutritional supplements. These options can provide results equivalent to or greater than those of conventional medicine without the unwanted side effects. In addition to the therapies discussed in this chapter, chiropractic and spinal manipulation,[34] craniosacral therapy,[35] biofeedback,[36] and massage[37] have all shown potential benefit. Most are not well served by clinical trials, but these therapies have many supporters who claim anecdotal effectiveness. If and when these therapies are subjected to sufficient clinical studies, I expect many of them will be shown to provide migraine relief.

Physical therapies provide a generally safe approach to migraine prevention and can be combined with nutritional supplementation and dietary modification. While these safe approaches to treatment and prevention offer advantages compared to conventional treatment, they will not be effective in all cases. People for whom these measures are not fully effective can consider drug-based solutions as a last resort.

CHAPTER 9

GET YOUR LIFE BACK

What we need is not the will to believe
but the will to find out.
—BERTRAND RUSSELL (1872–1970)

One of the main problems in dealing with nutrients and migraine is that few clinical trials have been conducted. According to recent medical conventions, randomized clinical trials are considered critical to the evaluation of potential treatments. However, although migraine is one of the most debilitating diseases on the planet, conventional medicine has generally failed to investigate the use of nutrition for prevention and treatment. Such neglect is strange, as nutritional triggers play a recognized part in the disease process.

This does not mean that migraineurs have no way to find treatments that are helpful to them. A migraine patient needs to take control of their disease and the healing process. Relying on doctors may delay or even prevent a successful outcome. Since migraine sufferers differ, each person will need to experiment to find what gives them the greatest relief with fewest side effects. Generally, this depends on the use of vitamins and other supplements rather than drugs. Some people find it useful to keep a diary in order to help identify their own migraine triggers and to record the effects of different treatments.

PREVENTION STEPS

It might seem an obvious first step to suggest that you avoid

143

migraine triggers and stressors. However, this is easier said than done. Individuals vary in their migraine triggers, and what leads to a migraine on a Monday may be different from that on a Saturday. Saturday migraine is well recognized, for example, and may be a response to the reduction in stress at the end of a busy working week.

Because of the complex nature of the condition, attempts to identify and avoid migraine triggers often result in little benefit, unless you keep a detailed diary of headaches and potential triggers over a long period of time, even years. Also, the apparent association between the "trigger" and the headache may be misleading. A person who has a headache after eating a bar of chocolate on Monday night might be responding to monosodium glutamate (MSG) in the Chinese dim sum he had on Sunday. It may appear from the diary that the chocolate is causing the headache, but the link could be deceptive. The difficulty is to determine the true triggers. Migraineurs generally have sufficient incentive to avoid the stressors that trigger their migraines and do not need to be reminded to do so.

Before you start experimenting, it is a good idea keep a diary for two or three months (longer if your migraines are infrequent). This is so you have a baseline against which to compare the effects of any supplements you try. Similar baselines are used by scientific researchers in migraine trials. It may be more practical to have as a "baseline" the previous therapy you investigated; that is, you can compare the effectiveness of two treatments. Record the number of migraines, how long they last, and the severity of pain or suffering. Women who might be suffering from menstrual migraines should also record when they have their period. Recording too many factors, such as bedtime, duration of sleep, and intake of various foods will not be helpful. The positive associations found by recording many factors will often occur by chance alone. Determining triggers with any degree of confidence using a diary is difficult.

Templates for diaries (of varying degrees of complexity) are readily available on the Internet: search for "migraine diary" and then choose one that makes sense and that you feel able to complete. You can alter the templates to fit your own situation. Remember, a simple diary will be both more practical and useful. Using a diary to investigate a migraine trigger is more effective and accurate if you have good reasons to believe that particular trigger causes migraines before you experiment.

MIGRAINE-PREVENTIVE THERAPIES

Throughout this book, it has been shown that vitamins and supplements provide the starting point for migraine prevention. In some cases, absorption of oral supplements can be limited, so it is a good idea to check with your health food shop or provider if there is any doubt. Nutrient supplements are generally safe and can be taken together. A little care may be needed with herbs, however, as they can produce side effects.

The supplements and strategies in the following list are in approximate order of benefit. So, those at the head of the list, such as magnesium and zinc, may be more likely to provide relief, or carry less risk of side effects, than those farther down. However, because of individual variation, this ranking is unlikely to be very accurate for any particular person.

You may choose to start with magnesium and zinc, for about four months, keeping a record in your migraine diary so you will be able to tell how much benefit you have obtained. Some fortunate individuals will respond well to magnesium and zinc and may not need additional supplementation. For others, magnesium and zinc may provide insufficient relief, so they might add the avoidance of dietary excitotoxins to their regimen. The combination of magnesium, zinc, plus no excitotoxins is more likely to be effective than magnesium and zinc alone.

By trying the therapies in sequence, the migraine sufferer can gain information about controlling their particular illness. For some, even the full combination of supplements, diet, and behavior change will provide limited benefit. In such cases, go back through the book, looking for other supplements that may provide benefit but which have limited or no support from clinical trials. Just because trials have not been carried out does not mean that particular substance will not work for you.

The fact that nutritional supplements are not being tested for their effects on migraine reflects a bias in the heart of medical science. Do not let the prejudice of conventional physicians, who should know better, cause you to continue suffering.

Magnesium and Zinc

As mentioned previously, magnesium injections can be used to abort a migraine attack. However, for prevention, oral supplements of magnesium are a useful option. The basic mechanisms of action are known and supported by physiological principles. To prevent migraines, start with a dose of approximately 100 mg of magnesium per day. Choose an easily absorbable form, such as magnesium chloride or magnesium malate. Do not take magnesium oxide, a cheap form that is not well absorbed, and avoid magnesium citrate and chelated magnesium, as they can contain aspartic acid, an excitotoxin and migraine trigger. Similarly, magnesium aspartate may precipitate migraine.

Make sure to check from the label that the tablet contains 100 mg of magnesium and that this weight applies to the magnesium element alone and does not include the chloride, for example. Gradually, increase the dose to near your maximum tolerable intake (the largest dose that does not cause loose stools or abdominal discomfort). Dividing the dose into two or three portions a day allows a greater intake than taking it all at once. The ability to absorb magnesium may change with time. For this reason, if you ever have gastrointestinal discomfort or loose stools, you should lower the dose to make sure you are not too near the maximum. Conversely, if you are constipated, you can probably increase your dose.

It takes time to alleviate a magnesium deficiency. Even if you are supplementing at close to bowel tolerance, it may take weeks to provide the maximum migraine prevention benefit. This is where your diary comes in handy, as it helps to compare how many migraines you had before and after the treatment.

Migraineurs also need to ensure that they are not deficient in zinc, otherwise they may not achieve the maximum benefit from the magnesium. However, while an adequate intake is beneficial, too great an intake of zinc can increase the chance of brain cell damage. An intake of 15 mg a day is the U.S. Recommended Dietary Allowance (RDA) and, for once, this seems a reasonable approximate intake. Consider 15–25 mg of zinc per day in an easily absorbable form.

Many people achieve a large reduction in migraine attacks with this nutrient combination. Even those who do not may reduce the number or severity of attacks and will be protecting their brain. This combination is a low-cost approach and provides additional health benefits.

Avoiding Excitotoxins

Even the most effective damping down of the migraine cycle will probably be ineffective against specific triggers. Excitotoxins are a hidden trigger found in many foods and drinks. Diet sodas contain aspartame and Chinese food is laced with monosodium glutamate: these are likely to invoke an attack in susceptible individuals, no matter what preventative measures are taken. Moreover, glutamate is often hidden in foods, where it is described as "hydrolyzed vegetable protein," "yeast extract," "malt extract," "flavoring" or "natural flavoring," and so on.

Take time to check the ingredients, especially on processed foods and drinks, and avoid exposure to excitotoxins. As a rule, avoid sugar substitutes, MSG, and related flavorings. This low-cost approach avoids junk food and provides added health benefits.

Curcumin and Boswellia

Curcumin, a derivative of turmeric, may be the most effective approach to migraine prevention and treatment. While writing this book, my experiments with highly absorbable forms of curcumin have provided greater relief than any other therapy. Curcumin is not at the top of this list because there are no clinical trials of curcumin in migraines. When the trials are performed, I would anticipate that absorbable curcumin will be the treatment of choice for migraine. Turmeric provides substantial health benefits and prevents many degenerative diseases, such as cancer and arthritis. Unfortunately, there are no long-term studies of the safety of curcumin derivatives at high doses. It is likely to be safe and generally prevent disease, but it is possible that some people will be sensitive to side effects. Personally, I am willing to take this small risk for the large benefits and relief of migraine that curcumin provides.

I have found the BCM-95 form of curcumin to be highly effective in preventing migraines. Moreover, the effect seems to occur rapidly, taking only a few days to develop. To be effective, it needs to be taken in repeated doses, perhaps three to four times each day. Curcumin (as standardized turmeric extract) is available in tablets of 250 mg, 500 mg, and 1,000 mg. A suggested initial intake for migraine prophylaxis is 500 mg of curcumin, twice a day. Take curcumin in absorbable form (e.g., BCM-95) and with a fish oil supplement, which will help assimilation.

Natural inflammation inhibitors are also found in boswellia, or its derivative 5-Loxin. While no direct trials have been conducted on these substances, they are considered safe and have a mechanism of action complementary to that of standard nonsteroidal drugs, such as naproxen or aspirin. Boswellia, or 5-Loxin, inhibits inflammation with a different mechanism of action to curcumin. The combination of curcumin and boswellia may be a particularly effective natural anti-inflammatory agent. A suggested dose is 250 mg of boswellia or 75 mg of 5-Loxin.

A high-dose vitamin C supplement (1 gram or more) is also recommended when taking these supplements. Turmeric extracts are relatively cheap. However, BCM-95 is currently more expensive, though the increased cost is offset by its enhanced efficacy. Perhaps the cost of this new form will lower with time.

Riboflavin and B-Complex Vitamins

A high-dose multiple B-vitamin, such as "B-100," will probably contain 100 mg of riboflavin, together with the supporting B-complex vitamins. A single B-100 supplement each day is suggested. Slow-release formulations will increase the amount of riboflavin absorbed. In trials, riboflavin has been effective in preventing migraine. Since the trials generally use a single daily dose of riboflavin, the amount absorbed is low. Thus, the benefits of riboflavin may have been grossly underestimated. To achieve the maximum benefit, take riboflavin four to six times per day in a relatively low dose (30 mg or more), in addition to the B-100. This is a low-cost approach and B-vitamin supplementation should be part of every healthy person's daily routine.

Melatonin

Melatonin is listed above coenzyme Q_{10} on this list partly because it costs less. Taken at night, melatonin helps stabilize the sleep-wake cycle; it is a powerful antioxidant and has been reported to prevent migraines. For migraine prophylaxis, high doses may be necessary. Any individual needs to find their most effective dose—for some, a low dose will be effective and higher doses will not be well tolerated; others will find benefit at higher intakes.

One approach is to start at a low dose, such as 1 mg taken thirty minutes before going to bed. Remain at this dose while monitoring your migraine attacks for at least a week. If the dose is not effective, increase it and monitor yourself for improvement and for increased daytime fatigue, which can be a side effect. Some people need doses of up to 20 mg each night to be effective against migraines. It is also worth noting that tolerance to melatonin can develop.

Ultimately, the aim is to find and take the lowest dose that provides the maximum benefit, without causing daytime fatigue. This is a low-cost approach.

Coenzyme Q_{10}

Coenzyme Q_{10} (CoQ_{10}) seems to prevent migraines. However, studies have been limited and may underestimate the effect. CoQ_{10} is a safe supplement and can be taken in high doses; its main "side effect" is improved health. The major limitation on using high doses of CoQ_{10} is the cost. It is also a little difficult to absorb orally. To improve absorption, take CoQ_{10} with fish oil. Some people also take CoQ_{10} with bioperine, a derivative of black pepper; this can increase absorption but may act indiscriminately, increasing absorption of some drugs, for example. The generally observed safe level of CoQ_{10}

is 1,200 mg and doses up to 3,000 mg per day are reported to be safe, so the question often becomes: how much can you afford? This is a higher-cost approach.

Fish Oil

Fish oil or omega-3 fatty acids may be helpful in preventing migraines. Omega-3s can inhibit inflammation and provide numerous additional health benefits (like many of the nutritional supplements discussed here). Taking fish oils together with fat-soluble vitamins and supplements may increase the absorption of these nutrients. It is sensible, for example, to combine a CoQ_{10} tablet with fish oil.

Be sure to use good-quality fish oils. Fish oil comes in capsule and liquid form. A 1,000-mg capsule might contain 400 mg of EPA (eicosapentaenoic acid) and 200 mg of DHA (docosahexaenoic acid). Once opened, fish oils oxidize quite quickly at room temperature, so they should be stored in an airtight container in the refrigerator. A typical starting intake for preventing migraine is three to five 1-gram capsules per day. This is a low-cost approach.

Ginger

Ginger is a particularly useful nutrient for both preventing and treating migraine. Since ginger is widely available and most people think it has a fantastic taste, it seems a great approach. Ginger may cause minor gastric upset but this is temporary and harmless. Try taking gram-level doses of dried ginger in capsules. Alternatively, hot infusions made with ginger root are most palatable. Ginger is inexpensive and high intakes in food or supplements can be safely consumed for long periods.

Feverfew

While feverfew has long been reported to prevent migraines and other headaches, how it achieves this effect is not established. Feverfew is an anti-inflammatory and prevents blood platelets sticking together. Either of these actions could explain how it prevents migraines. Feverfew extract is available in several forms and suggested doses. Although dried feverfew leaves are obtainable, and fresh ones may grow in your garden, it may be tricky to adjust dosage with these. Standardized products are offered, containing 0.5–1.0 percent parthenolide. A typical tablet size is 100–400 mg and the recommended frequency varies from one to six tablets a day, with meals. Try starting at a low dose (a single daily tablet) and increase to the maximum recommended intake, if necessary. As with any of these preventative measures, it may take up to four months to achieve benefit.

Make sure you are aware of the possible drug interactions and side effects, particularly allergic reactions. Side effects may include abdominal pain, flatulence, diarrhea, indigestion, nausea, vomiting, and nervousness. Chewing the leaves can lead to temporary loss of taste and swelling of the mouth. Take particular care if you are allergic to chamomile, ragweed, or yarrow. These potential issues mean herbs such as feverfew are intermediate between the safety of nutrients and the less desirable effects of drugs. This is a low-cost approach.

Alpha-Lipoic Acid and Acetyl-L-Carnitine

While there are no clinical trials on the combination of alpha-lipoic acid and acetyl-L-carnitine, there are theoretical reasons to think it may help prevent migraines. Also, in my experience, they are helpful both in preventing attacks and in lowering their intensity. These nutrients are available as separate supplements or combined in a single tablet. The sodium or potassium salt of R-alpha-lipoic acid is the preferred form of lipoic acid. Typical recommended doses are 100 mg of alpha-lipoic acid and 500 mg of acetyl-L-carnitine, four times a day. This is a medium-cost approach.

Glucosamine and Chondroitin

In addition to curcumin and boswellia, glucosamine and chondroitin can alleviate inflammation and prevent migraine. These anti-inflammatory supplements have an excellent safety record and are widely available, as they are often used in combination with fish oils to prevent arthritis. Glucosamine and chondroitin provide another alternative to nonsteroidal anti-inflammatory drugs (NSAIDs) for controlling inflammation and migraine headaches. A typical combination tablet may contain 500 mg of glucosamine and 100 mg of chondroitin. These should be taken two to three times a day. Glucosamine and chondroitin supplements are relatively cheap.

5-Hydroxytryptophan (5-HTP)

Many migraineurs report 5-HTP is useful at preventing migraines. It is available in tablets, typically taken in the range 50–100 mg per day. Check with your physician for any potential drug interactions and follow the advice of the manufacturer. Start taking one tablet and increase to about 300 mg per day in divided doses.

Kava-Kava

Kava-kava is a controversial supplement but it may help prevent migraine. There are some concerns about rare side effects, particularly liver damage. Some countries, such as Canada, have banned the sale of this herb. However, other scientists dispute the connection with liver damage.[1] Until 1998, kava was considered safe and free of side effects. The problem may have arisen as a result of companies preparing poor-quality herb in alcohol or acetone.[2] Notably, kava is sold as a relaxant and tranquilizer and thus potentially competes with several highly profitable drugs. This herb does not agree with me, but other people have found it exceptionally helpful. It is not available for sale in all countries, but those who find the risk acceptable can obtain it via the Internet. A typical dose is 250 mg one to three times a day, but it may not be suitable for continuous use. Once again, check with your physician about its use and any drug interactions. Kava is a low-cost solution.

Tips on Prevention

A preventative treatment may take three to four months before maximum benefit is achieved. This presents the migraineur looking for a way to overcome the illness with a dilemma. It cannot be determined in advance which preventative treatment will work; it is necessary to try possible preventions over a long period. Each treatment should be compared with background or baseline information before starting the therapy to see whether a good response is due to the treatment.

Every potential treatment needs to be tried alone, although a new one can be added to an existing therapeutic regimen. That is, if you have a baseline using magnesium, zinc, and curcumin, then the benefit of adding riboflavin to the mix can be checked. But in order to have a reasonable idea which combination of supplements is providing optimal benefit, they each need to be tested.

A particular treatment may initially have good prevention results but might then tail off with use. You can exploit this phenomenon by changing a preventative therapy from time to time. Typically, it takes two to four months for a treatment to become fully effective. So, changing potential treatments every six months may be helpful. A possible sequence might be ginger followed by glucosamine, which then changes to 5-HTP, and so on. Try leaving a gap of three months before returning to a treatment.

There is no simple solution to preventing migraine in all cases. However, vitamin and mineral supplements are often as effective as the most powerful drugs available. In addition, they will help prevent other illnesses and maintain good health. A person using supplements can always use conventional medical approaches in addition to supplements, if necessary, to improve chances of having fewer migraines.

MIGRAINE-ABORTIVE THERAPIES

When migraine prevention fails, which is possible with any preventative approach, the immediate treatment aim should be to abort the attack. The earlier that action is taken, the more effective the treatment is likely to be. The following short list covers some natural options for aborting migraine attacks. These remedies do not have major side effects. Although the list avoids options likely to interfere with the use of migraine-abortive drugs, it is important to check the side effects and interactions with any conventional drug before using it. If in doubt about the side effects of a drug or its interactions, seek advice from a doctor or pharmacist.

Keeping a Cool Head

Lowering the temperature of the head is a non-invasive and safe migraine therapy, which can provide relief or even abort an attack. Specific anti-migraine headgear provides an alternative to the ice pack approach. Try an ice pack to relieve your headache and you may find it provides adequate relief or, at least, reduces your intake of analgesics (such as NSAIDs) and other abortive drugs (such as triptans). Head cooling caps have a relatively high initial cost but may prove cost-effective if used over a longer period.

Niacin

If taken early, niacin (vitamin B_3) can abort a migraine. Niacin causes acute skin flushing, which seems to be necessary to abort the attack. A relatively large dose (500–1,000 mg) may provide rapid relief from the headache. Andrew Saul, Ph.D., suggests 500 mg every half hour at the start of an attack, until a flush is achieved. Being used to the flushing effect, I find that a single large dose (1,000 mg) brings on an intense flush more quickly and is more likely to be effective. Niacin is an inexpensive supplement.

Curcumin

Curcumin can be a highly effective migraine abortant, provided it is absorbed well. The low absorption rate of oral curcumin normally limits its use in migraine and inflammation. Taking curcumin sublingually, or in liposomal form, can provide sufficient absorption to abort a migraine attack. I have found that 400 mg of the BCM-95 form can rapidly abort a migraine if taken sublingually and held in the mouth. The beneficial effect can be dramatic. Alternatively, a larger dose (2–5 grams) of BCM-95 taken orally takes two to four hours to be effective. Absorbable curcumin (BCM-95) is not expensive compared with triptan drugs.

Ginger

Taken in the prodrome phase, ginger may prevent an attack before it really gets started. During an attack, it helps prevent nausea and allow absorption from the stomach and intestines. Ginger capsules are readily available (500 mg is a common size). At the start of an attack, I would likely take three to five capsules to preserve stomach absorption. A proprietary combination of ginger and feverfew, taken sublingually, has also been used to abort a migraine headache. In addition to adding ginger to food or using supplements, crystallized ginger can be helpful. Normally, I avoid sugar and refined carbohydrates whenever possible. However, carbohydrates can be useful early in a migraine attack and occasionally abort it. Ginger is a low-cost solution that provides a good excuse for eating candy.

Vitamin B_{12}

Vitamin B_{12} (typically a 5-mg tablet), taken sublingually, can ease the pain of a migraine. Vitamin B_{12} inhibits nitric oxide and can lower the inflammation and blood vessel dilation that occurs in a migraine. In my experience, 5 mg of sublingual B_{12} has about the same effect as an aspirin—not enough to abort a migraine but it does provide a little help.

Vitamin C

Massive doses of vitamin C can get someone through an otherwise unbearable migraine attack. It will not stop the pain but it may make it more tolerable. Do not take more than 2 grams at a time unless you know your bowel tolerance levels, otherwise you could suffer a laxative effect. Vitamin C needs to be taken early. Large quantities— 5 to 10 grams or more per day in divided doses—may be necessary.

Liposomal vitamin C is particularly effective at improving well-being and may be absorbed even during an attack.

Oxygen

Breathing oxygen can provide relief for migraine attacks. While oxygen is not commonly available, it deserves a mention because it may be tried when drugs are ineffective. Oxygen therapy is relatively safe.

Transcranial Magnetic Stimulation and Acupuncture

Physical therapies, such as transcranial magnetic stimulation (TMS) and acupuncture, are increasingly used for aborting a migraine. However, an acupuncturist may not be immediately available when an attack occurs, so this approach may be more suitable for migraine prevention. TMS is in its early stages of development with an uncertain safety profile.

Magnesium Injections

Magnesium injections are a recognized, if controversial, approach to relieving migraine attacks. Try to convince your physician that injections of magnesium sulfate can be a safe approach to aborting a severe migraine. For some people, magnesium sulfate injections may provide both rapid relief from a severe migraine and a period of freedom from the disease, as it restores the body's magnesium levels. People can also be trained to give themselves injections. However, such injections should not be too frequent. This is not a method for preventing migraines—it should be reserved for ending acute attacks, as recommended by a physician. Liposomal magnesium, when available, could provide an alternative to injections in aborting migraines.

CONCLUSION

Targeted treatment requires an accurate diagnosis—it is therefore essential to give your doctor a full account of all your symptoms. Headache is a non-specific symptom and is common to many illnesses. However, a person with a history of headache with nausea or vomiting, especially if the pain is throbbing and affects one side of the head, is likely to have migraines.

Conventional medicine has not served migraine sufferers well. The current fashion demands statistical evidence from large trials. Despite this, the requisite placebo-controlled, double-blind, large-scale clinical trials have not been conducted for many nutritional migraine treatments. Direct supporting evidence and smaller studies do exist, but may not find their way into the mainstream medical literature. Your doctor may not be aware of this research, as I found when asking for magnesium injections. Safe magnesium therapy has been ignored by the medical mainstream, which favors profit-making anti-migraine drugs, regardless of possible side effects. Often, pharmaceutical researchers attempt to emulate the action of nutrients, such as magnesium (NMDA-receptor blockers) or turmeric (novel anti-inflammatories).

Nutritional treatments are generally safer than drug therapy and can be at least as effective. Nevertheless, migraine sufferers are likely to find that physicians tend to stick to accepted medical practice and can be overly cautious about trying nutritional therapies. Conservatism is not necessarily a bad attribute in a medic: in the case of drugs, it is a good idea to be wary, as many have side effects. However, if the treatments in question are nutrients, then the risks are minimal. By definition, nutrients are part of the diet, have few side effects, and can be consumed with a high degree of safety. For a migraine sufferer, the risk associated with failing to test preventative or curative nutrients is much higher than the likelihood of suffering a side effect. By not trying nutritional treatments, you risk losing all the days you might otherwise have been free of symptoms. This is clearly a substantial risk!

Vitamins and nutritional treatments are mostly cheap and safe, and evidence from clinical trials suggests they are at least as effective as conventional treatments and drugs. The limited trials on vitamin B_2 (riboflavin) and CoQ_{10} (CoQ_{10}) indicate that these nutrients' effectiveness in preventing migraines is equivalent to current drug treatment. The evidence for magnesium's anti-migraine effect is particularly strong: injected magnesium sulfate will abort a migraine attack. Unfortunately, rather than ensuring migraine sufferers are not deficient in magnesium, the conventional medical/pharmaceutical response has been to copy the action of this essential mineral in a drug therapy (memantine).

The influence of diet on migraine is widely accepted, though conventional medicine emphasizes negative effects (triggers). It is widely believed that dietary substances, such as monosodium glutamate (MSG) or chocolate, may cause headaches; doctors commonly advise their patients to remove offending triggers from their diet. Other dietary modifications, such as lowering carbohydrate intake, can also prevent attacks, though these are not standard medical practice. The assumption that dietary components have a purely one-sided action—in other words, that nutrients can increase but not decrease the number of migraine attacks—is illogical.

Migraine treatments are not limited to painkillers and associated drugs. Vitamins and other nutrients provide an optimal combination of effectiveness and safety, and should be the first line of attack for the treatment of migraines. Physical therapies, including head cooling and acupuncture, can also provide benefit. Changes in behavior, such as avoiding bright sunshine, are understandable, once it is realized that migraine attacks occur through a positive feedback loop. Avoiding triggers is another behavioral approach, but the problem

is to find out which triggers affect you. Even when triggers are eliminated, the disease may adjust and other causative agents come into
play. Removing excitotoxins (such as MSG) and other common
offenders provides an effective and simple approach to preventing
migraines.

An experimental approach to the use of vitamins and other supplements, as well as physical therapies and lifestyle changes, can help
you develop an effective therapy for your migraines, allowing you
to reclaim your life and well-being. Since standard medical advice
excludes many helpful approaches, migraineurs need to take respon-
sibility for their own treatment. Failure to do this may result in years
of suffering.

REFERENCES

Introduction

1. World Health Organization (WHO). *Neurological Disorders, Public Health Challenges*. Geneva, Switzerland: WHO, 2006.

2. World Health Organization (WHO). *Mental Health: New Understanding, New Hope*. Geneva, Switzerland: WHO, 2001, pp. 22–24.

3. Stovner, L.J., K. Hagen, R. Jensen, et al. "The Global Burden of Headache: A Documentation of Headache Prevalence and Disability Worldwide." *Cephalalgia* 27:3 (2007): 193–210.

4. Stovner, L.J., and K. Hagen. "Prevalence, Burden and Cost of Headache Disorders." *Curr Opin Neurol* 19 (2006): 281–285.

5. Lipton, R.B., M.E. Bigal, K. Kolodner, et al. "The Family Impact of Migraine: Population-based Studies in the U.S. and U.K." *Cephalalgia* 23 (2003): 429–440.

6. Steiner, T.J., A.I. Scher, W.F. Stewart, et al. "The Prevalence and Disability Burden of Adult Migraine in England and Their Relationships to Age, Gender and Ethnicity." *Cephalalgia* 23 (2003): 519–527.

Chapter 1: The Migraine Experience

1. Phillips, H. "Is Migraine All in the Mind?" *New Scientist* (June 21, 2003): 36–39.

2. Steiner, T.J., A.I. Scher, W.F. Stewart, et al. "The Prevalence and Disability Burden of Adult Migraine in England and Their Relationships to Age, Gender and Ethnicity." *Cephalalgia* 23 (2003): 519–527.

3. Miranda, H., G. Ortiz, S. Figueroa, et al. "Prevalence of Headache in Puerto Rico." *Headache* 43 (2003): 774–778. Morillo, L.E., F. Alarcon, N. Aranaga, et al. "Prevalence of Migraine in Latin America." *Headache* 45 (2005): 106–117.

4. Celik, Y., G. Ekuklu, B. Tokuç, et al. "Migraine Prevalence and Some Related Factors in Turkey." *Headache* 45 (2005): 32–36.

5. Lipton, R.B., W.F. Stewart, S. Diamond, et al. "Prevalence and Burden of Migraine in the United States: Data from the American Migraine Study II." *Headache* 41:7 (2001): 646–657.

6. Headache Classification Subcommittee of the International Headache Society. "The International Classification of Headache Disorders." *Cephalalgia* 24:Suppl 1 (2004): 1–160.

7. Couturier, E.G., M.A. Bomhof, A.K. Neven, et al. "Menstrual Migraine in a Representative Dutch Population Sample: Prevalence, Disability and Treatment." *Cephalalgia* 23:4 (2003): 302–308. Granella, F., G. Sances, G. Allais, et al. "Characteristics of Menstrual and Nonmenstrual Attacks in Women with Menstrually Related Migraine Referred to Headache Centres." *Cephalalgia* 24:9 (2004): 707–716.

8. Ferrari, M.D. "Migraine." *Lancet* 351 (1998): 1043–1051.

9. Edmeads, J. "The Treatment of Headache: A Historical Perspective." In Gallagher, R.M. (ed.). *Therapy for Headache.* New York: Marcel Dekker, 1990.

10. Unger, J. "Migraine Headaches: A Historical Prospective, a Glimpse into the Future, and Migraine Epidemiology." *Dis Mon* 52:10 (2006): 367–384.

11. Wolf, G. "A Historical Note on the Mode of Administration of Vitamin A for the Cure of Night Blindness." *Am J Clin Nutr* 31 (1978): 290–292.

12. Headache Classification Subcommittee of the International Headache Society. "The International Classification of Headache Disorders." *Cephalalgia* 24:Suppl 1 (2004): 1–160.

13. Hopkins, A. "Neurological Services and the Neurological Health of the Population in the United Kingdom." *J Neurol Neurosurg Psychiatry* 63:Suppl 1 (1997): S53–S59.

14. Lipton, R.B., A.I. Scher, T.J. Steiner, et al. "Patterns of Health Care Utilization for Migraine in England and in the United States." *Neurology* 60 (2003): 441–448.

15. Schreiber, C., S. Hutchinson, C. Webster, et al. "Prevalence of Migraine in Patients with a History of Self-reported or Physician-diagnosed 'Sinus' Headache." *Arch Intern Med* 164:16 (2004): 1769–1772. Mehle, M.E., and C.P. Schreiber. "Sinus Headache, Migraine, and the Otolaryngologist." *Otolaryngol Head Neck Surg* 133:4 (2005): 489–496.

16. Ishkanian, G. "Efficacy of Sumatriptan Tablets in Migraineurs Self-described or Physician-diagnosed as Having Sinus Headache: A Randomized, Double-blind, Placebo-controlled Study." *Clin Ther* 29:1 (2007): 99–109.

17. Vincent, M.B., and N. Hadjikhani. "Migraine Aura and Related Phenomena: Beyond Scotomata and Scintillations." *Cephalalgia* 27:12 (2007): 1368–1377.

18. Santoro, G., B. Casadei, A. Venco. "The Transient Global Amnesia-Migraine Connection, Case Report." *Funct Neurol* 3:3 (1988): 353–360. Crowell, G.F., D.A. Stump, J. Biller, et al. "The Transient Global Amnesia-Migraine Connection." *Arch Neurol* 41:1 (1984): 75–79.

19. Chambliss, J., M. Cook, D. Williams, et al. "Painting Dreams Shaped by Epilepsy and the Auras of Migraines." *J Clin Neurosci* 15:3 (2008): 360.

20. Unger, J. "Migraine Headaches: A Historical Prospective, a Glimpse into the Future, and Migraine Epidemiology." *Dis Mon* 52:10 (2006): 367–384. Jones, J.M. "Great Pains: Famous People with Headaches." *Cephalalgia* 19:7 (1999): 627–630.

21. Rogawski, M.A. "Common Pathophysiologic Mechanisms in Migraine and Epilepsy." *Arch Neurol* 65:6 (2008): 709–714.

22. Lauritzen, M. "Pathophysiology of the Migraine Aura. The Spreading Depression Theory." *Brain* 117:Part 1 (1994): 199–210.

23. Didion, J. *The White Album*. New York: Farrar, Straus and Giroux, 1990.

24. Phillips, H. "Is Migraine All in the Mind?" *New Scientist* (June 21, 2003): 36–39.

25. Didion, J. *The White Album*. New York: Farrar, Straus and Giroux, 1990.

26. Society for the Advancement of Education. "Migraine: Pain is So Severe, 'I've Wished I Were Dead'." *USA Today Special Newsletter Edition: Your Health* (October 1994).

27. Pietrobon, D. "Familial Hemiplegic Migraine." *Neurotherapeutics* 4:2 (2007): 274–284.

28. Edvinsson, L., and R. Uddman. "Neurobiology in Primary Headaches." *Brain Res Brain Res Rev* 48:3 (2005): 438–456.

29. Loder, E. "What Is the Evolutionary Advantage of Migraine?" *Cephalalgia* 22 (2002): 624–632.

Chapter 2: A Search for Causes

1. Kirsch, I., B.J. Deacon, T.B. Huedo-Medina, et al. "Initial Severity and Anti-depressant Benefits: A Meta-Analysis of Data Submitted to the Food and Drug Administration." *PLoS Med* 5:2 (2008): e45.

2. Edvinsson, L., and R. Uddman. "Neurobiology in Primary Headaches." *Brain Res Brain Res Rev* 48:3 (2005): 438–456.

3. Lambert, G.A., and A.S. Zagami. "The Mode of Action of Migraine Triggers: A Hypothesis." *Headache* 49:2 (2009): 253–275.

4. Burstein, R., and M. Jakubowski. "Unitary Hypothesis for Multiple Triggers of the Pain and Strain of Migraine." *J Comp Neurol* 493:1 (2005): 9–14.

5. Swaminathan, N. "Blood Flow May Be Key Player in Neural Processing." *Sci Am* (January 24, 2008).

6. Aurora, S.K., and K.M. Welch. "Migraine: Imaging the Aura." *Curr Opin Neurol* 13:3 (2000): 273–276.

7. Huth, E.J., and T.J. Murray. *Medicine in Quotations.* Philadelphia: ACP Press, 2006, p. 260.

8. Drubach, D. *The Brain Explained.* Upper Saddle River, NJ: Prentice Hall, 1999.

9. Wolf, S. "In Memoriam Harold G. Wolff, M.D." *Psychosomatic Med* 24:3 (1962): 222–224.

10. Mauskop, A., and B. Fox. *What Your Doctor May Not Tell You About Migraines.* New York: Grand Central Publishing, 2001.

11. Dalessio, D.J. "Vascular Permeability and Vasoactive Substances: Their Relationship to Migraine." *Adv Neurol* 4 (1974): 395–401. Dalessio, D.J. "A Classification of Headache." *Int Ophthalmol Clin* 10 (1970): 647–665. Moskowitz, M.A. "The Neurobiology of Vascular Head Pain." *Ann Neurol* 2 (1984): 157–168.

12. Tfelt-Hansen, P, P.R. Saxena, C. Dahlöf, et al. "Ergotamine in the Acute Treatment of Migraine: A Review and European Consensus." *Brain* 123:Part 1 (2000): 9–18.

13. Kangasniemi, P., and C. Hedman. "Metoprolol and Propranolol in the Prophylactic Treatment of Classical and Common Migraine. A Double-blind Study." *Cephalalgia* 4:2 (2002): 91–96. Ramadan, N.M. "Current Trends in Migraine Prophylaxis." *Headache* 47:Suppl 1 (2007): S52–S57.

14. Schoenen, J. (1986) "Beta Blockers and the Central Nervous System." *Cephalalgia* 6:Suppl 5 (1986): 47–54.

15. Bahra, A., M.S. Matharu, C. Buchelb, et al. "Brainstem Activation Specific to Migraine Headache." *Lancet* 357:9261 (2001): 1016–1017.

16. Schoonman, G.G., J. van der Grond, C. Kortmann, et al. "Migraine Headache Is Not Associated with Cerebral or Meningeal Vasodilation—A 3T Magnetic Resonance Angiography Study." *Brain* 131:8 (2008): 2192–2200.

17. Bahra, A., M.S. Matharu, C. Buchelb, et al. "Brainstem Activation Specific to Migraine Headache." *Lancet* 357:9261 (2001): 1016–1017. May, A., A. Bahra, C. Buchel, et al. "Hypothalamic Activation in Cluster Headache Attacks." *Lancet* 352 (1998): 275–278. May, A., C. Buchel, R. Turner, et al. "MR-Angiography in Facial and Other Pain: Neurovascular Mechanisms of Trigeminal Sensation." *J Cereb Blood Flow Metab* 21 (2001): 1171–1176. May, A., C. Buchel, R. Turner, et al. "Neurovascular Dilatation of Intracranial Vessels in Experimental Headache." *Cephalalgia* 19 (1999): 464–465.

18. Sicuteri, F. "Headache Biochemistry and Pharmacology." *Arch Neurobiol* 37 (1974): 27–65.

19. Waeber, C., and M.A. Moskowitz. "Migraine as an Inflammatory Disorder." *Neurology* 64:Suppl 2 (2005): S9–S15.

20. Peroutka, S.J. "Neurogenic Inflammation and Migraine: Implications for the Therapeutics." *Mol Interv* 5:5 (2005): 304–311.

21. Longoni, M., and C. Ferrarese. "Inflammation and Excitotoxicity: Role in Migraine Pathogenesis." *Neurol Sci* 27 (2006): S107–S110.

22. Moskowitz, M.A. "The Neurobiology of Vascular Head Pain." *Ann Neurol* 16 (1984): 157–168. Markowitz, S., K. Saito, M.A. Moskowitz. "Neurogenically Mediated Leakage of Plasma Protein Occurs from Blood Vessels in Dura Mater but Not Brain." *J Neurosci* 7 (1987): 4129–4136.

23. Puri, V., S. Puri, S.R. Svojanovsky, et al. "Effects of Oestrogen on Trigeminal Ganglia in Culture: Implications for Hormonal Effects on Migraine." *Cephalalgia* 26:1 (2006): 33–42.

24. Buzzi, M.G., and M.A. Moskowitz. "The Anti-migraine Drug, Sumatriptan (GR43175), Selectively Blocks Neurogenic Plasma Extravasation from Blood Vessels in Dura Mater." *Br J Pharmacol* 99 (1990): 202–206.

25. Saito, K., S. Markowitz, M.A. Moskowitz. "Ergot Alkaloids Block Neurogenic Extravasation in Dura Mater: Proposed Action in Vascular Headache." *Ann Neurol* 24 (1988): 732–737.

26. Goadsby, P.J., and L. Edvinsson. "The Trigeminovascular System and Migraine: Studies Characterizing Cerebrovascular and Neuropeptide Changes Seen in Humans and Cats." *Ann Neurol* 33 (1993): 48–56.

27. Holzer, P. "Neurogenic Vasodilatation and Plasma Leakage in the Skin." *Gen Pharmacol* 1 (1998): 5–11.

28. Lassen, L.H., P.A. Haderslev, V.B. Jacobsen, et al. "CGRP May Play a Causative Role in Migraine." *Cephalalgia* 22:1 (2002): 54–61.

29. Fox, F.E., M. Kubin, M. Cassin, et al. "Calcitonin Gene–related Peptide Inhibits Proliferation and Antigen Presentation by Human Peripheral Blood Mononuclear Cells: Effects on B7, Interleukin 10, and Interleukin 12." *J Invest Dermatol* 108 (1997): 43–48.

30. Goadsby, P.J. and L. Edvinsson. "The Trigeminovascular System and Migraine: Studies Characterizing Cerebrovascular and Neuropeptide Changes Seen in Humans and Cats." *Ann Neurol* 33 (1993): 48–56.

31. Durham, P.L.. and A.F. Russo. "Regulation of Calcitonin Gene–related Peptide Secretion by a Serotonergic Antimigraine Drug." *J Neurosci* 19:9 (1999): 3423–3429.

32. Xiao, Y., J.A. Richter, J.H. Hurley. "Release of Glutamate and CGRP from Trigeminal Ganglion Neurons: Role of Calcium Channels and 5-HT1 Receptor Signaling." *Mol Pain* 4 (2008): 12.

33. Link, A.S., A. Kuris, L. Edvinsson. "Treatment of Migraine Attacks Based

on the Interaction with the Trigemino-cerebrovascular System." *J Headache Pain* 9:1 (2008): 5–12.

34. Olesen, J., H. Diener, I.W. Husstedt, et al., and the BIBN 4096 BS Clinical Proof of Concept Study Group. "Calcitonin Gene–related Peptide Receptor Antagonist BIBN 4096 BS for the Acute Treatment of Migraine." *N Engl J Med* 350:11 (2004): 1104–1110. Arulmani, U., A. Maassenvandenbrink, C.M. Villalón, et al. "Calcitonin Gene–related Peptide and Its Role in Migraine Pathophysiology." *Eur J Pharmacol* 500:1–3 (2004): 315–330.

35. Edvinsson, L. "Clinical Data on the CGRP Antagonist BIBN4096BS for Treatment of Migraine Attacks." *CNS Drug Rev* 11:1 (2005): 69–76.

36. Blaylock, R.L. *Excitotoxins: The Taste That Kills.* Santa Fe, NM: Health Press, 1996.

37. Montagna, P., T. Sacquegna, P. Cortelli, et al. "Migraine as a Defect of Brain Oxidative Metabolism: A Hypothesis." *J Neurol* 236:2 (1989): 124–125.

38. Klopstock, T., A. May, P. Seibel, et al. "Mitochondrial DNA in Migraine with Aura." *Neurology* 46 (1996): 1735–1738.

39. Porter, A., J.P. Gladstone, D.W. Dodick. "Migraine and White Matter Hyperintensities." *Curr Pain Headache Rep* 9:4 (2005): 289–293. Speciali, J.G., and M.E. Bigal. "Subcortical Lesions in Migraine: Are They Related to Mitochondrial Dysfunction?" *Headache* 46:9 (2006): 1461–1462.

40. Fukuhara, N., S. Tokiguchi, K. Shirakawa, et al. "Myoclonus Epilepsy Associated with Ragged-red Fibers (Mitochondrial Abnormalities): Disease Entity or a Syndrome? Light-and Electron-Microscopic Studies of Two Cases and Review of Literature." *J Neurol Sci* 47:1 (1980): 117–133.

41. Melone, M.A., A. Tessa, S. Petrini, et al. "Revelation of a New Mitochondrial DNA Mutation (G12147A) in a MELAS/MERFF Phenotype." *Arch Neurol* 61:2 (2004): 269–272.

42. Sangiorgi, S., M. Mochi, R. Riva, et al. "Abnormal Platelet Mitochondrial Function in Patients Affected by Migraine with and without Aura." *Cephalalgia* 14:1 (2002): 21–23.

43. Klopstock, T., A. May, P. Seibel, et al. "Mitochondrial DNA in Migraine with Aura." *Neurology* 46 (1996): 1735–1738.

44. Granziera, C., A.F.M. DaSilva, J. Snyder, et al. "Anatomical Alterations of the Visual Motion Processing Network in Migraine with and without Aura." *PLoS Med* 3:10 (2006): e402.

45. DaSilva, A.F., C. Granziera, J. Snyder, et al. "Thickening in the Somatosensory Cortex of Patients with Migraine." *Neurology* 69:21 (2007): 1990–1995.

46. Swaab, D.F., E.J. Dubelaar, M.A. Hofman, et al. "Brain Aging and Alzheimer's Disease; Use It or Lose It." *Prog Brain Res* 138 (2002): 343–373.

47. Wilkins, A.J. *Visual Stress.* London: Oxford University Press, 1995.

48. Fernandez, D., and A.J. Wilkins. "Uncomfortable Images in Art and Nature." *Perception* 37:7 (2008): 1098–1113.

49. Dobson R. "What Pain Looks Like." *The Independent* (January 13, 2009): 12–13.

50. Wiener, N. *Cybernetics: Control and Communication in the Animal and the Machine.* Cambridge, MA: The MIT Press, 1948.

51. Le Fanu, J. *The Rise and Fall of Modern Medicine.* Jackson, TN: Basic Books, 2002.

52. American Academy of Neurology. "Is It All In Your Head? No, Weather Can Trigger Migraines." *Science Daily* (January 25, 2000).

53. Bell, I.R., E.E. Hardin, C.M. Baldwin, et al. "Increased Limbic System Symptomatology and Sensitizability of Young Adults with Chemical and Noise Sensitivities." *Environ Res* 70:2 (1995): 84–97.

54. De Marinis, M., A. Pujia, E. Colaizzo, et al. "The Blink Reflex in 'Chronic Migraine'." *Clin Neurophysiol* 118:2 (2007): 457–463.

55. Sacks, O. *Migraine.* London: Vintage, 1999.

56. Millichap, J.G., and M.M. Yee. "The Diet Factor in Pediatric and Adolescent Migraine." *Pediatr Neurol* 28:1 (2003): 9–15.

57. Ibid.

58. Monro, A.A. "Food Allergy in Migraine." *Proc Nutr Soc* 42 (1983): 241–246.

59. Egger, J., J. Wilson, C.M. Carter, et al. "Is Migraine Food Allergy? A Double-blind Controlled Trial of Oligoantigenic Diet Treatment." *Lancet* 322:8355 (1983): 865–869.

60. Egger, J., C.M. Carter, J.F. Soothill, et al. "Oligoantigenic Diet Treatment of Children with Epilepsy and Migraine." *J Pediatr* 114:1 (1989): 51–58.

61. Mansfield, L.E., T.R. Vaughan, S.F. Waller, et al. "Food Allergy and Adult Migraine: Double-blind and Mediator Confirmation of an Allergic Etiology." *Ann Allergy* 55:2 (1985): 126–129.

62. Arroyave Hernández, C.M., M. Echevarría Pinto, H.L. Hernández Montiel. "Food Allergy Mediated by IgG Antibodies Associated with Migraine in Adults." *Rev Alerg Mex* 54:5 (2007): 162–168.

Chapter 3: Diagnosing a Migraine

1. "International Classification of Headache Disorders, 2nd Edition." *Cephalalgia* 24:Suppl 1 (2004): 9–160.

2. Rasmussen, B.K. "Epidemiology of Headache." *Cephalalgia* 15 (1995): 45–68.

3. Beck, E., W.J. Sieber, R. Trejo. "Management of Cluster Headache." *Am Fam Physician* 71:4 (2005): 717–724.

4. Mauskop, A., B.T. Altura, R.Q. Cracco, et al. "Intravenous Magnesium Sulfate Relieves Cluster Headaches in Patients with Low Serum Ionized Magnesium Levels." *Headache* 35:10 (1995): 597–600.

5. Mauskop, A., B.T. Altura, R.Q. Cracco, et al. "Intravenous Magnesium Sulfate Rapidly Alleviates Headaches of Various Types." *Headache* 36:3 (1996): 154–160.

6. Bahra, A., M. Walsh, S. Menon, et al. "Does Chronic Daily Headache Arise De Novo in Association with Regular Use of Analgesics?" *Headache* 43:3 (2003): 179–190.

7. Goadsby, P.J., and C. Boes. "Chronic Daily Headache." *J Neurol Neurosurg Psychiatry* 72:Suppl 2 (2002): ii2–ii5.

8. Castillo, J., et al. "Epidemiology of Chronic Daily Headache in the General Population." *Headache* 39 (1999): 190–196. Srikiatkhachorn, A., and K. Phanthurachinda. "Prevalence and Clinical Features of Chronic Daily Headache in a Headache Clinic." *Headache* 37 (1997): 277–280.

9. Eross, E.J. "Chronic Migraine and Medication-overuse Headache." *Neurology* 66 (2006): E43–E44.

10. Diener, H.C., J. Dichgans, E. Scholz, et al. "Analgesic-induced Chronic Headache: Long-term Results of Withdrawal Therapy." *J Neurol* 236 (1989): 9–14.

11. World Health Organization (WHO). *Neurological Disorders, Public Health Challenges.* Geneva, Switzerland: WHO, 2006.

12. Goadsby, P.J., and C. Boes. "Chronic Daily Headache." *J Neurol Neurosurg Psychiatry* 72:Suppl 2 (2002): ii2–ii5.

13. American Association for the Study of Headache and International Headache Society. "Consensus Statement on Improving Migraine Management." *Headache* 38 (1998): 736.

14. Limmroth, V., Z. Kazarawa, G. Fritsche, et al. "Headache after Frequent Use of Serotonin Agonists Zolmitriptan and Naratriptan." *Lancet* 353 (1999): 378. Bateman, D.N. "Triptans and Migraine." *Lancet* 355:9207 (2000): 860–861.

15. Duarte, R.A., and D.R. Thornton. "Short-acting Analgesics May Aggravate Chronic Headache Pain." *Am Fam Physician* 51 (1995): 203.

16. Schnider, P., et al. "Long-term Outcome of Patients with Headache and Drug Abuse after Inpatient Withdrawal: Five-year Follow-up." *Cephalalgia* 16 (1996): 481–485.

17. Hering, R., and T.J. Steiner. "Abrupt Outpatient Withdrawal of Medication in Analgesic-abusing Migraineurs." *Lancet* 337 (1991): 1442–1443.

18. Schnider, P., et al. "Long-term Outcome of Patients with Headache and Drug Abuse after Inpatient Withdrawal: Five-year Follow-up." *Cephalalgia* 16 (1996): 481–485.

19. Clissold, S.P. "Paracetamol and Phenacetin." *Drugs* 32:Suppl 4 (1986): 46–59.

20. Lee, W.M. "Acetaminophen and the U.S. Acute Liver Failure Study Group: Lowering the Risks of Hepatic Failure." *Hepatology* 40:1 (2004): 6–9.

21. McLean, A.E., and P.A. Day. "The Effect of Diet on the Toxicity of Paracetamol and the Safety of Paracetamol-Methionine Mixtures." *Biochem Pharmacol* 24:1 (1975): 37–42. Skoglund, L.A., K. Ingebrigtsen, P. Lausund, et al. "Plasma Concentration of Paracetamol and Its Major Metabolites after P. O. Dosing with Paracetamol or Concurrent Administration of Paracetamol and Its N-Acetyl- DL-Methionine Ester in Mice." *Gen Pharmacol* 23 (1992): 155–158.

22. Crome, P., G.N. Volans, R. Goulding, et al. "Oral Methionine in the Treatment of Severe Paracetamol (Acetaminophen) Overdose." *Lancet* 2 (1976): 829–830. Hamlyn, A.N., M. Lesna, C.O. Record, et al. "Methionine and Cysteamine in Paracetamol (Acetaminophen) Overdose, Prospective Controlled Trial of Early Therapy." *J Int Med Res* 9 (1981): 226–231. Prescott, L.F., J. Park, G.R. Sutherland, et al. "Cysteamine, Methionine, and Penicillamine in the Treatment of Paracetamol Poisoning." *Lancet* 2 (1976): 109–113.

23. Alsalim, W., and M. Fadel. "Oral Methionine Compared with Intravenous N-Acetyl Cysteine for Paracetamol Overdose." *Emerg Med J* 20:4 (2003): 366–367.

24. Frishberg, B.M., et al. *Evidence-based Guidelines in the Primary Care Setting: Neuroimaging in Patients with Nonacute Headache.* Saint Paul, MN: American Academy of Neurology, 2001. Castillo, J., et al. "Epidemiology of Chronic Daily Headache in the General Population." *Headache* 39 (1999): 190–196.

25. Ophoff, R.A., G.M. Terwindt, M.N. Vergouwe, et al. "Familial Hemiplegic Migraine and Episodic Ataxia Type-2 are Caused by Mutations in the Ca^{2+} Channel Gene CACNL1A4." *Cell* 87:3 (1996): 543–552.

26. Thomsen, L.L., E. Ostergaard, J. Olesen, et al. "Evidence for a Separate Type of Migraine with Aura: Sporadic Hemiplegic Migraine." *Neurology* 60:4 (2003): 595–601.

27. Lykke, T.L., E.M. Kirchmann, R.S. Faerch, et al. "An Epidemiological Survey of Hemiplegic Migraine." *Cephalalgia* 22:5 (2002): 361–375.

28. Victor, M., A.H. Ropper, R.D. Adams. *Adams and Victor's Principles of Neurology,* 7th revised edition. New York: McGraw-Hill, 2001.

29. Haan, J., G.M. Terwindt, R.A. Ophoff, et al. for the Dutch Migraine Genetics Research Group. "Is Familial Hemiplegic Migraine a Hereditary Form of Basilar Migraine?" *Cephalalgia* 15:6 (2002): 477–481.

30. Classification Subcommittee of the International Headache Society. "The International Classification of Headache Disorders." *Cephalalgia* 24:Suppl 1 (2004): 9–160. Russell, G., I. Abu-Arafeh, D.N. Symon. "Abdominal Migraine: Evidence for Existence and Treatment Options." *Paediatr Drugs* 4:1 (2002): 1–8.

31. Fazekas, F., M. Koch, R. Schmidt, et al. "The Prevalence of Cerebral Damage Varies with Migraine Type: A MRI Study." *Headache* 32:6 (1992): 287–291.

32. Evans, R.W. "New Daily Persistent Headache." *Curr Pain Headache Rep* 7:4 (2003): 303–307. Nahab, F.B., G.A. Worrell, B.G. Weinshenker. "25-Year-Old Man with Recurring Headache and Confusion." *Mayo Clin Proc* 76 (2001): 75–78.

33. Frishberg, B.M., et al. *Evidence-based Guidelines in the Primary Care Setting: Neuroimaging in Patients with Nonacute Headache.* Saint Paul, MN: American Academy of Neurology, 2001.

34. Darkeh, A.K. "Glaucoma, Acute Angle-Closure." WebMD, http://emedicine.medscape.com/article/798811-overview (article updated August 12, 2009).

35. Tang, H., and J.H.K. Ng. "Googling for a Diagnosis—Use of Google as a Diagnostic Aid: Internet Based Study." *Br Med J* 333 (2006): 1143–1145. Editor. "Google is a Good Diagnostician." *Br Med J* 333 (December 2, 2006).

Chapter 4: Avoid Junk Food

1. Rogawski, M.A. "Common Pathophysiologic Mechanisms in Migraine and Epilepsy." *Arch Neurol* 65:6 (2008): 709–714.

2. Gursoy-Ozdemir, Y., J. Qiu, N. Matsuoka, et al. "Cortical Spreading Depression Activates and Regulates MMP-9." *J Clin Invest* 113 (2004): 1447–1455.

3. Scheller, D., S. Szathmary, J. Kolb, et al. "Observations on the Relationship between the Extracellular Changes of Taurine and Glutamate during Cortical Spreading Depression, during Ischemia, and within the Area Surrounding a Thrombotic Infarct." *Amino Acids* 19 (2000): 571–583. Lauritzen, M., and A.J. Hansen. "The Effect of Glutamate Receptor Blockade on Anoxic Depolarization and Cortical Spreading Depression." *J Cereb Blood Flow Metab* 12 (1992): 223–229.

4. Hill, R.G., and T.E. Salt. "An Ionophoretic Study of the Responses of Rat Caudal Trigeminal Nucleus Neurons to Non-noxious Mechanical Sensory Stimuli." *J Physiol* 327 (1982): 65–78. Bereiter, D.A., and A.P. Benetti. "Excitatory Amino Acid Release within Spinal Trigeminal Nucleus after Mustard Oil Injection into the Temporomandibular Joint Region of the Rat." *Pain* 67 (1996): 451–459.

5. Bolay, H., U. Reuter, A.K. Dunn, et al. "Intrinsic Brain Activity Triggers Trigeminal Meningeal Afferents in a Migraine Model." *Nat Med* 8:2 (2002): 136–142.

6. Trauba, R., Y. Jia, B. Tanga. "Estrogen Increases NMDA Receptor Expression and Phosphorylation Modulating Visceral Pain in the Rat." *J Pain* 8:4 Suppl 1 (2007): S14. Gureviciene, I., J. Puoliväli, R. Pussinen, et al. "Estrogen Treatment Alleviates NMDA-antagonist Induced Hippocampal LTP Blockade and Cognitive Deficits in Ovariectomized Mice." *Neurobiol Learn Mem* 79:1 (2003): 72–80.

7. Foy, M.R., J. Xu, X. Xie, et al. "17Beta-Estradiol Enhances NMDA Receptor-mediated EPSPs and Long-term Potentiation." *J Neurophysiol* 81:2 (1999): 925–929.

8. Kwok, R.H.M. "The Chinese Restaurant Syndrome." *N Engl J Med* 278 (1968): 796.

9. Schaumburg. H.H., R. Byck, R. Gerstl, et al. "Monosodium L-Glutamate: Its Pharmacology and Role in the Chinese Restaurant Syndrome." *Science* 163:869 (1969): 826–828.

10. Kenney, R.A. "The Chinese Restaurant Syndrome: An Anecdote Revisited." *Food Chem Toxicol* 24:4 (1986): 351–354. Tarasoff, L., and M.F. Kelly. "Monosodium L-Glutamate: A Double-blind Study and Review." *Food Chem Toxicol* 31:12 (1993): 1019–1035.

11. Freeman, M. "Reconsidering the Effects of Monosodium Glutamate: A Literature Review." *J Am Acad Nurse Pract* 18:10 (2006): 482–486. Geha, R.S., A. Beiser, C. Ren, et al. "Review of Alleged Reaction to Monosodium Glutamate and Outcome of a Multicenter Double-blind Placebo-controlled Study." *J Nutr* 130:4S Suppl (2000): 1058S–1062S.

12. Vikelis, M., and D.D. Mitsikostas. "The Role of Glutamate and Its Receptors in Migraine." *CNS Neurol Disord Drug Targets* 6:4 (2007): 251–257. Ramadan, N.M. "The Link between Glutamate and Migraine." *CNS Spectr* 8:6 (2003): 446–449.

13. Blaylock, R.L. *Excitotoxins: The Taste That Kills.* Santa Fe, NM: Health Press, 1996.

14. Gobatto, C.A., M.A. Mello, C.T. Souza, et al. "The Monosodium Glutamate (MSG) Obese Rat as a Model for the Study of Exercise in Obesity." *Res Commun Mol Pathol Pharmacol* 111:1–4 (2002): 89–101.

15. Hermanussen, M., A.P. García, M. Sunder, et al. "Obesity, Voracity, and Short Stature: The Impact of Glutamate on the Regulation of Appetite." *Eur J Clin Nutr* 60:1 (2006): 25–31.

16. Harper, A.M., E.T. MacKenzie, J. McCulloch, et al. "Migraine and the Blood-Brain Barrier." *Lancet* 1:8020 (1977): 1034–1036.

17. Hargreaves, R.J., and S.L. Shepheard. "Pathophysiology of Migraine—New Insights." *Can J Neurol Sci* 26:Suppl 3 (1999): S12–S19.

18. Dziedzic, J. "Are White Matter Lesions a Plausible Risk Factor for Migraine?" *NeurologyReviews.com.* 15:4 (April 2007).

19. Sachdev, P., W. Wen, X. Chen, et al. "Progression of White Matter Hyper-intensities in Elderly Individuals Over 3 Years." *Neurology* 68:3 (2007): 214–222.

20. Kruit, M.C., M.A. van Buchem, P.A. Hofman, et al. "Migraine as a Risk Factor for Subclinical Brain Lesions." *JAMA* 291:4 (2004): 427–434. Swartz, R.H., and R.Z. Kern. "Migraine Is Associated with Magnetic Resonance Imaging White Matter Abnormalities: A Meta-analysis." *Arch Neurol* 61:9 (2004): 1366–1368.

21. Ramadan, N.M. "The Link between Glutamate and Migraine." *CNS Spectr* 8:6 (2003): 446–449.

22. Cananzi, A.R., G. D'Andrea, F. Perini, et al. "Platelet and Plasma Levels of Glutamate and Glutamine in Migraine with and without Aura." *Cephalalgia* 15:2 (1995): 132–135. Ferrari, M.D., J. Odink, K.D. Bos, et al. "Neuroexcitatory Plasma Amino Acids Are Elevated in Migraine." *Neurology* 40:10 (1990): 1582–1586. Alam, Z., N. Coombes, R.H. Waring, et al. "Plasma Levels of Neuroexcitatory Amino Acids in Patients with Migraine or Tension Headache." *J Neurol Sci* 156:1 (1998): 102–106. D'Andrea, G., A.R. Cananzi, R. Joseph, et al. "Platelet Glycine, Glutamate and Aspartate in Primary Headache." *Cephalalgia* 11:4 (1991): 197–200.

23. Martinez, F., J. Castillo, J.R. Rodriguez, et al. "Neuroexcitatory Amino Acid Levels in Plasma and Cerebrospinal Fluid during Migraine Attacks." *Cephalalgia* 13 (1993): 89–93.

24. Rothrock, J.F., K.R. Mar, T.L. Yaksh, et al. "Cerebrospinal Fluid Analyses in Migraine Patients and Controls." *Cephalalgia* 15:6 (1995): 489–493.

25. Martinez, F., J. Castillo, J.R. Rodriguez, et al. "Neuroexcitatory Amino Acid Levels in Plasma and Cerebrospinal Fluid during Migraine Attacks." *Cephalalgia* 13 (1993): 89–93.

26. Castillo, J., F. Martinez, R. Leira, et al. "Changes in Neuroexcitatory Amino Acids during and between Migraine Attacks." *Neurologia* 9:2 (1994): 42–45.

27. Longoni, M., and C. Ferrarese. "Inflammation and Excitotoxicity: Role in Migraine Pathogenesis." *Neurol Sci* 27 (2006): S107–S110.

28. Koehler, S.M., and A. Glaros. "The Effect of Aspartame on Migraine Headache." *Headache* 28:1 (1988): 10–14. Lipton, R.B., L.C. Newman, J.S. Cohen, et al. "Aspartame as a Dietary Trigger of Headache." *Headache* 29:2 (1989): 90–92.

29. Stegink, L.D, L.J. Filer, E.F. Bell, et al. "Plasma Amino Acid Concentrations in Normal Adults Administered Aspartame in Capsules or Solution: Lack of Bioequivalence." *Metabolism* 36:5 (1987): 507–512. Stegink, L.D, L.J. Filer, G.L. Baker. "Plasma Amino Acid Concentrations in Normal Adults Ingesting Aspartame and Monosodium L-Glutamate as Part of a Soup/Beverage Meal." *Metabolism* 36:11 (1987): 1073–1079.

30. Olney, J.W. "Excitotoxins in Foods." *Neurotoxicology* 15:3 (1994): 535–544.

31. Reynolds, W.A., V. Butler, N. Lemkey-Johnston. "Hypothalamic Morphology Following Ingestion of Aspartame or MSG in the Neonatal Rodent and Primate: A Preliminary Report." *J Toxicol Environ Health* 2:2 (1976): 471–480.

32. González-Quevedo, A., F. Obregón, M. Urbina, et al. "Effect of Chronic Methanol Administration on Amino Acids and Monoamines in Retina, Optic Nerve, and Brain of the Rat." *Toxicol Appl Pharmacol* 185:2 (2002): 77–84.

33. Blumenthal, H.J., and D.A. Vance. (1997) "Chewing Gum Headaches." *Headache* 37:10 (1997): 665–666.

34. Newman, L.C., and R.B. Lipton. "Migraine MLT-down: An Unusual Presentation of Migraine in Patients with Aspartame-triggered Headaches." *Headache* 41:9 (2001): 899–901.

35. Johns, D.R. "Migraine Provoked by Aspartame." *N Engl J Med* 315:7 (1986): 456.

36. Butchko, H.H., W.W. Stargel, C.P. Comer, et al. "Aspartame: Review of Safety." *Regul Toxicol Pharmacol* 35:2 Part 2 (2002): S1–S93.

37. Olney, J.W. "Excitotoxins in Foods." *Neurotoxicology* 15:3 (1994): 535–544. Whitehouse, C.R., J. Boullata, L.A. McCauley. "The Potential Toxicity of Artificial Sweeteners." *AAOHN J* 56:6 (2008): 251–259.

38. Walton, R.G. "Survey of Aspartame Studies: Correlation of Outcome and Funding Sources." (1998.) Available online at: www.dorway.com. Accessed December 26, 2008.

39. Artis. A.M. Letter to Martini, B.L., from the Department of Health and Human Services, U.S. Food and Drug Administration, June 6, 1996.

40. Strong, F.C. "Why Do Some Dietary Migraine Patients Claim They Get Headaches from Placebos?" *Clin Exp Allergy* 30:5 (2000): 739–743.

41. Strong, F.C. "It May Be the Caffeine in Extra Strength Excedrin that is Effective for Migraine." *J Pharm Pharmacol* 49:12 (1997): 1260.

42. Blaylock, R.L. *Excitotoxins: The Taste That Kills.* Santa Fe, NM: Health Press, 1996.

43. Maizels, M., A. Blumenfeld, R. Burchette. "A Combination of Riboflavin, Magnesium, and Feverfew for Migraine Prophylaxis: A Randomized Trial." *Headache* 44:9 (2004): 885–890.

44. Zempleni, J., J.R. Galloway, D.B. McCormick. "Pharmacokinetics of Orally and Intravenously Administered Riboflavin in Healthy Humans." *Am J Clin Nutr* 63:1 (1996): 54–66.

45. Mathew, S.J., K. Keegan, L. Smith. "Glutamate Modulators as Novel Interventions for Mood Disorders." *Rev Bras Psiquiatr* 27:3 (2005): 243–248.

46. Phelps, L.E., N. Brutsche, J.R. Moral, et al. "Family History of Alcohol Dependence and Initial Antidepressant Response to an N-methyl-D-aspartate Antagonist." *Biol Psychiatry* 65:2 (2009): 181–184.

47. Mathew, S.J., K. Keegan, L. Smith. "Glutamate Modulators as Novel Interventions for Mood Disorders." *Rev Bras Psiquiatr* 27:3 (2005): 243–248.

48. Decollogne, S., A. Tomas, C. Lecerf, et al. "NMDA Receptor Complex Blockade by Oral Administration of Magnesium: Comparison with MK-801." *Pharmacol Biochem Behav* 58:1 (1997): 261–268.

49. Szewczyk, B., E. Poleszak, M. Sowa-Kucma, et al. "Antidepressant Activity of Zinc and Magnesium in View of the Current Hypotheses of Antidepressant Action." *Pharmacol Rep* 60:5 (2008): 588–589.

50. Sucher, N.J., and S.A. Lipton. "Redox Modulatory Site of the NMDA Receptor-channel Complex: Regulation by Oxidized Glutathione." *J Neurosci Res* 30:3 (1991): 582–591. Choi, Y.B., and S.A. Lipton. "Redox Modulation of the NMDA Receptor." *Cell Mol Life Sci* 57:11 (2000): 1535–1541.

51. Aizenman, E., S.A. Lipton, R.H. Loring. "Selective Modulation of NMDA Responses by Reduction and Oxidation." *Neuron* 2:3 (1989): 1257–1263.

52. Levy, D.I., N.J. Sucher, S.A. Lipton. "Redox Modulation of NMDA Receptor-mediated Toxicity in Mammalian Central Neurons." *Neurosci Lett* 110:3 (1990): 291–296.

53. Ibid.

54. Dawson, V.L., T.M. Dawson, D.A. Bartley, et al. "Mechanisms of Nitric Oxide–mediated Neurotoxicity in Primary Brain Cultures." *J Neurosci* 13:6 (1993): 2651–2661.

55. Williams, L.R. "Oxidative Stress, Age-related Neurodegeneration, and the Potential for Neurotrophic Treatment." *Cerebrovasc Brain Metab Rev* 7:1 (1995): 55–73. Lipton, S.A., and P. Nicotera. "Calcium, Free Radicals and Excitotoxins in Neuronal Apoptosis." *Cell Calcium* 23:2–3 (1998): 165–171. Pellegrini-Giampietro, D.E., G. Cherici, M. Alesiani, et al. "Excitatory Amino Acid Release and Free Radical Formation May Cooperate in the Genesis of Ischemia-induced Neuronal Damage." *J Neurosci* 10:3 (1990): 1035–1041.

Chapter 5: Preventing a Migraine with Nutrition

1. Atkins, R.C. *Dr. Atkins' New Diet Revolution.* New York: M. Evans, 2003.

2. Banting, W. *Letter on Corpulence.* New York: Cosimo Classics, 2005.

3. Brunton, L., J. Lazo, K. Parker. *Goodman and Gilman's The Pharmacological Basis of Therapeutics.* New York: McGraw-Hill, 2005.

4. Freeman, J.M., E.H. Kossoff, A.L. Hartman. "The Ketogenic Diet: One Decade Later." *Pediatrics* 119:3 (2007): 535–543. Neal, E.G., H. Chaffe, R.H. Schwartz, et al. "The Ketogenic Diet for the Treatment of Childhood Epilepsy: A Randomised Controlled Trial." *Lancet Neurol* 7:6 (2008): 500–506.

5. Levy, R., and P. Cooper. "Ketogenic Diet for Epilepsy." *Cochrane Database Syst Rev* 1 (2005): CD001903.

6. Neal, E.G., H. Chaffe, R.H. Schwartz, et al. "The Ketogenic Diet for the Treatment of Childhood Epilepsy: A Randomised Controlled Trial." *Lancet Neurol* 7:6 (2008): 500–506.

7. National Institute for Clinical Excellence (NICE). "CG20 Epilepsy in Adults and Children: Full Guideline." London: NICE, October 2004.

8. Sirven, J., B. Whedon, D. Caplan, et al. "The Ketogenic Diet for Intractable Epilepsy in Adults: Preliminary Results." *Epilepsia* 40:12 (1999): 1721–1726. Kim do, Y., and J.M. Rho. "The Ketogenic Diet and Epilepsy." *Curr Opin Clin Nutr Metab Care* 11:2 (2008): 113–120.

9. Freeman, J.M., E.H. Kossoff, A.L. Hartman. "The Ketogenic Diet: One Decade Later, State-of-the-Art Review Article." *Pediatrics* 119:3 (2007): 535–543. Strahlman, R.S. "Can Ketosis Help Migraine Sufferers? A Case Report." *Headache* 46:1 (2006): 182.

10. Yudkoff, M., Y. Daikhin, I. Nissim, et al. "Ketogenic Diet, Brain Glutamate Metabolism and Seizure Control." *Prostaglandins Leukot Essent Fatty Acids* 70:3 (2004): 277–285. Daikhin, Y., and M. Yudkoff. "Ketone Bodies and Brain Glutamate and GABA Metabolism." *Dev Neurosci* 20:4–5 (1998): 358–364.

11. Blaylock, R.L. *Excitotoxins: The Taste That Kills.* Santa Fe, NM: Health Press, 1996.

12. Hickey, S., and H. Roberts "Selfish Cells: Cancer as Microevolution." *J Orthomolecular Med* 23:3 (2006): 137–146.

13. Weitzman, S. "Alternative Nutritional Cancer Therapies." *Int J Cancer Suppl* 11 (1998): 69–72.

14. Vaughan, T.R. "The Role of Food in the Pathogenesis of Migraine Headache." *Clin Rev Allergy* 12:2 (1994): 167–180.

15. Nelson, H.S., J. Oppenheimer, A. Buchmeier, et al. "An Assessment of the Role of Intradermal Skin Testing in the Diagnosis of Clinically Relevant Allergy to Timothy Grass." *J Allergy Clin Immunol* 97:6 (1996): 1193–1201. Bousquet, J., B. Lebel, H. Dhivert, et al. "Nasal Challenge with Pollen Grains, Skin-prick Tests and Specific IgE in Patients with Grass Pollen Allergy." *Clin Allergy* 17:6 (1987): 529–536.

16. Hickey, S., H.J. Roberts, R.F. Cathcart. "Dynamic Flow." *J Orthomolecular Med* 20:4 (2005): 237–244.

17. Ilhan, A., E. Uz, A. Var, et al. "Diagnostic Role of Hair Magnesium in Migraine Patients: Higher Than Serum Magnesium?" *Trace Elements Electrolytes* 17:1 (2000): 14–18.

18. Blaylock, R.L. *Excitotoxins: The Taste That Kills.* Santa Fe, NM: Health Press, 1996.

19. Mauskop, A., and B.M. Altura. "Role of Magnesium in the Pathogenesis and Treatment of Migraines." *Clin Neurosci* 5:1 (1998): 24–27.

20. Schoenen, J., J. Sianard-Gainko, M. Lenaerts. "Blood Magnesium Levels in Migraine." *Cephalalgia* 11:2 (2002): 97–99. Gallai, V., P. Sarchielli, G. Coata, et al. "Serum and Salivary Magnesium Levels in Migraine. Results in a Group of Juvenile Patients." *Headache* 32:3 (2005): 132–135.

21. Ramadan, N.M., H. Halvorson, A. Vande-Linde, et al. "Low Brain Magnesium in Migraine." *Headache* 29:7 (1989): 416–419.

22. Welch, K.M., and N.M. Ramadan. "Mitochondria, Magnesium and Migraine." *J Neurol Sci* 134:1–2 (1995): 9–14.

23. Peikert, A., C. Wilimzig, R. Köhne-Volland. "Prophylaxis of Migraine with Oral Magnesium: Results from a Prospective, Multi-center, Placebo-controlled and Double-blind Randomized Study." *Cephalalgia* 16:4 (1996): 257–263.

24. Pfaffenrath, V., P. Wessely, C. Meyer, et al. "Magnesium in the Prophylaxis of Migraine—A Double-blind Placebo-controlled Study." *Cephalalgia* 16:6 (1996): 436–440.

25. Wang, F., S.K. Van Den Eeden, L.M. Ackerson, et al. "Oral Magnesium Oxide Prophylaxis of Frequent Migrainous Headache in Children: A Randomized, Double-blind, Placebo-controlled Trial." *Headache* 43:6 (2003): 601–610.

26. Mount, C., and C. Downton. "Alzheimer Disease: Progress or Profit?" *Nat Med* 12:7 (2006): 780–784.

27. Charles, A., C. Flippen, M. Romero Reyes, et al. "Memantine for Prevention of Migraine: A Retrospective Study of 60 Cases." *J Headache Pain* 8:4 (2007): 248–250.

28. Bigal, M., A. Rapoport, F. Sheftell, et al. "Memantine in the Preventive Treatment of Refractory Migraine." *Headache* 48:9 (2008): 1337–1342.

29. Frankiewicz, T., and C.G. Parsons. "Memantine Restores Long-term Potentiation Impaired by Tonic N-Methyl-D-Aspartate (NMDA) Receptor Activation Following Reduction of Mg2+ in Hippocampal Slices." *Neuropharmacology* 38:9 (1999): 1253–1259.

30. Offer, A. "The Cover-Up of Hidden MSG." *Natural News Newsletter* (December 12, 2008).

31. Donma, O., and M.M. Donma. "Association of Headaches and the Metals." *Biol Trace Elem Res* 90:1–3 (2002): 1–14.

32. Faden, A.I. "Liposome Entrapped Magnesium." European Patent Office, International Application PCT/US1988/001006, 1987.

33. Waring, R.H. "Report on Absorption of Magnesium Sulfate (Epsom Salts) Across the Skin." Epson Salt Council, www.epsomsaltcouncil.org, 2004. Available online at: http://www.epsomsaltcouncil.org/articles/Report_on_Absorption_of_magnesium_sulfate.pdf.

34. Smart, T.G., A.M. Hosie, P.S. Miller. "Zn²⁺ Ions: Modulators of Excitatory and Inhibitory Synaptic Activity." *Neuroscientist* 10:5 (2004): 432–442. Li, Y.V., C.J. Hough, J.M. Sarvey. "Do We Need Zinc to Think?" *Sci STKE* 182 (2003): 19.

35. Hollmann, M., J. Boulter, C. Maron, et al. "Zinc Potentiates Agonist-induced Currents at Certain Splice Variants of the NMDA Receptor." *Neuron* 10:5 (1993): 943–954.

36. Takeda, A., T. Hanajima, H. Ijiro, et al. "Release of Zinc from the Brain of El (Epilepsy) Mice During Seizure Induction." *Brain Res* 828:1–2 (1999): 174–178.

37. Takeda, A. "Zinc Homeostasis and Functions of Zinc in the Brain." *Biometals* 14:3–4 (2001): 343–351.

38. Weiss, J.H., S.L. Sensi, J.Y. Koh. "Zn(2+): A Novel Ionic Mediator of Neural Injury in Brain Disease." *Trends Pharmacol Sci* 21:10 (2000): 395–401.

39. Harrison, D.P. "Copper as a Factor in the Dietary Precipitation of Migraine." *Headache* 26:5 (1986): 248–250.

40. Harrison, D.P. "Migraine Headaches and Wilson's Disease Associated with Intrauterine Copper Contraceptive Devices." *Am J Optometry Physiol Optics* 62:8 (1985): 575–577.

41. Seaman, B., and G. Seaman. "Recovering from the Pill." In *Women and the Crisis in Sex Hormones*. New York: Rawson, 1977, pp. 109–133.

42. Grant, E.C.G. "The Pill, Hormone Replacement Therapy, Vascular and Mood Over-reactivity, and Mineral Imbalance." *J Nutr Environ Med* 8:2 (1998): 105–116.

43. Blaylock, R.L. *Excitotoxins: The Taste That Kills*. Santa Fe, NM: Health Press, 1996.

44. Rozen, T.D., M.L. Oshinsky, C.A. Gebeline, et al. "Open Label Trial of Coenzyme Q₁₀ as a Migraine Preventive." *Cephalalgia* 22:2 (2002): 137–141.

45. Zmitek, J., A. Smidovnik, M. Fir, et al. "Relative Bioavailability of Two Forms of a Novel Water-soluble Coenzyme Q₁₀." *Ann Nutr Metab* 52:4 (2008): 281–287.

46. Sándor, P.S., L. Di Clemente, G. Coppola, et al. "Efficacy of Coenzyme Q₁₀ in Migraine Prophylaxis: A Randomized Controlled Trial." *Neurology* 64:4 (2005): 713–715.

47. Hershey, A.D., S.W. Powers, A.L. Vockell, et al. "Coenzyme Q₁₀ Deficiency and Response to Supplementation in Pediatric and Adolescent Migraine." *Headache* 47:1 (2007): 73–80.

48. Silvestrini, M., M. Bartolini, M. Coccia, et al. "Topiramate in the Treatment of Chronic Migraine." *Cephalalgia* 23:8 (2003): 820–824. Storey, J.R.,

C.S. Calder, D.E. Hart, et al. "Topiramate in Migraine Prevention: A Double-blind, Placebo-controlled Study." *Headache* 41:10 (2001): 968–975.

49. Safety Officer in Physical Chemistry. "Safety Data for Coenzyme Q_{10}." MSDS Safety Sheet, Oxford University, March 2007.

50. Brody, T. *Nutritional Biochemistry*, 2nd Edition. San Diego, CA: Academic Press, 1999. U.S. Institute of Medicine. "Riboflavin." In *Dietary Reference Intakes: Thiamin, Riboflavin, Niacin, Vitamin B_6, Vitamin B_{12}, Pantothenic Acid, Biotin, and Choline.* Washington, DC: Food and Nutrition Board, National Academy Press, 1998.

51. Powers, H.J. "Current Knowledge Concerning Optimum Nutritional Status of Riboflavin, Niacin and Pyridoxine." *Proc Nutr Soc* 58:2 (1999): 435–440.

52. Ibid.

53. Jacques, P.F., A.G. Bostom, P.W. Wilson, et al. "Determinants of Plasma Total Homocysteine Concentration in the Framingham Offspring Cohort." *Am J Clin Nutr* 73:3 (2001): 613–621.

54. Wacker, J., J. Fruhauf, M. Schulz, et al. "Riboflavin Deficiency and Preeclampsia." *Obstet Gynecol* 96:1 (2000): 38–44.

55. Neugebauer, J., Y. Zanre, J. Wacker. "Riboflavin Supplementation and Preeclampsia." *Int J Gynaecol Obstet* 93:2 (2006): 136–137.

56. Schoenen, J., J. Jacquy, M. Lenaerts. "Effectiveness of High-dose Riboflavin in Migraine Prophylaxis: A Randomized Controlled Trial." *Neurology* 50:2 (1998): 466–470.

57. Boehnke, C., U. Reuter, U. Flach, et al. "High-dose Riboflavin Treatment Is Efficacious in Migraine Prophylaxis: An Open Study in a Tertiary Care Centre." *Eur J Neurol* 11:7 (2004): 475–477.

58. Magis, D., A. Ambrosini, P. Sándor, et al. "A Randomized Double-blind Placebo-controlled Trial of Thioctic Acid in Migraine Prophylaxis." *Headache* 47:1 (2007): 52–57.

59. Kabbouche, M.A., S.W. Powers, A.L. Vockell, et al. "Carnitine Palmityl-transferase II (CPT2) Deficiency and Migraine Headache: Two Case Reports." *Headache* 43:5 (2003): 490–495.

60. Hsu, C.C., Y.H. Chuang, J.L. Tsai, et al. "CPEO and Carnitine Deficiency Overlapping in MELAS Syndrome." *Acta Neurol Scand* 92:3 (1995): 252–255.

61. Peres, M.F. "Melatonin, the Pineal Gland and Their Implications for Headache Disorders." *Cephalalgia* 25:6 (2005): 403–411.

62. Dodick, D.W., and D.J. Capobianco. "Treatment and Management of Cluster Headache." *Curr Pain Headache Rep* 5:1 (2001): 83–91. Peres, M.F., M.R. Masruha, E. Zukerman, et al. "Potential Therapeutic Use of Melatonin in Migraine and Other Headache Disorders." *Expert Opin Investig Drugs* 15:4

(2006): 367–375. Peres, M.F., E. Zukerman, F. da Cunha Tanuri, et al. "Melatonin, 3 mg, Is Effective for Migraine Prevention." *Neurology* 63:4 (2004): 757.

63. Gagnier, J.J. "The Therapeutic Potential of Melatonin in Migraines and Other Headache Types." *Altern Med Rev* 6:4 (2001): 383–389.

64. Claustrat, B., C. Loisy, J. Brun, et al. "Nocturnal Plasma Melatonin Levels in Migraine: A Preliminary Report." *Headache* 29:4 (1989): 242–245.

65. Brun, J., B. Claustrat, P. Saddier, et al. "Nocturnal Melatonin Excretion Is Decreased in Patients with Migraine without Aura Attacks Associated with Menses." *Cephalalgia* 15:2 (1995): 136–139.

66. Murialdo, G., S. Fonzi, P. Costelli, et al. "Urinary Melatonin Excretion Throughout the Ovarian Cycle in Menstrually Related Migraine." *Cephalalgia* 14:3 (1994): 205–209.

67. Claustrat, B., J. Brun, M. Geoffriau, et al. "Nocturnal Plasma Melatonin Profile and Melatonin Kinetics During Infusion in Status Migrainosus." *Cephalalgia* 17:4 (1997): 511–517.

68. Nagtegaal, J.E., M.G. Smits, A.C. Swart, et al. "Melatonin-responsive Headache in Delayed Sleep Phase Syndrome: Preliminary Observations." *Headache* 38:4 (1998): 303–307.

69. Miano, S., P. Parisi, A. Pelliccia, et al. "Melatonin to Prevent Migraine or Tension-type Headache in Children." *Neurol Sci* 29:4 (2008): 285–287.

70. Zhdanova, I.V., R.J. Wurtman, M.M. Regan, et al. "Melatonin Treatment for Age-related Insomnia." *J Clin Endocrinol Metab* 86:10 (2001): 4727–4730.

71. Badia, P., R.J. Hughes, K.P. Wright, et al. "High-dose Melatonin Facilitates Sleep without Negative Carryover on Performance." *Sleep Res* 25 (1996): 541.

72. Clarke, J.R., B. Schultz, L. Crepeau, et al. "Evaluating the Effects of High-Dose Melatonin on Mental and Somatic Status of Normal Subjects." Washington, DC: Storming Media Pentagon Reports, A796244, 2003.

73. Shokouhi, G., R.S. Tubbs, M.M. Shoja, et al. "Neuroprotective Effects of High-dose vs. Low-dose Melatonin after Blunt Sciatic Nerve Injury." *Childs Nerv Syst* 24:1 (2008): 111–117. Ayer, R.E., T. Sugawara, W. Chen, et al. "Melatonin Decreases Mortality Following Severe Subarachnoid Hemorrhage." *J Pineal Res* 44:2 (2008): 197–204.

74. Kwok, B.H., B. Koh, M.I. Ndubuisi, et al. "The Anti-inflammatory Natural Product Parthenolide from the Medicinal Herb Feverfew Directly Binds To and Inhibits IkappaB Kinase." *Chem Biol* 8:8 (2001): 759–766.

75. Pittler, M.H., and E. Ernst. "Feverfew for Preventing Migraine." *Cochrane Database Syst Rev* (2004): CD002286.

76. Johnson, E.S., N.P. Kadam, D.M. Hylands, et al. "Efficacy of Feverfew as Prophylactic Treatment of Migraine." *Br Med J* 291:6495 (1985): 569–573.

77. Palevitch, D., G. Earon, R. Carasso. "Feverfew (*Tanacetum parthenium*) as a Prophylactic Treatment for Migraine: A Double-blind Placebo-controlled Study." *Phytotherapy Res* 11:7 (1998): 508–511.

78. Murphy, J.J., S. Heptinstall, J.R. Mitchell. "Randomised Double-blind Placebo-controlled Trial of Feverfew in Migraine Prevention." *Lancet* 2:8604 (1988): 189–192.

79. Diener, H.C., V. Pfaffenrath, J. Schnitker, et al. "Efficacy and Safety of 6.25 mg t.i.d. Feverfew CO_2-extract (MIG-99) in Migraine Prevention—A Randomized, Double-blind, Multicentre, Placebo-controlled Study." *Cephalalgia* 25:11 (2005): 1031–1041.

80. Yao, M., H.E. Ritchie, P.D. Brown-Woodman. "A Reproductive Screening Test of Feverfew: Is a Full Reproductive Study Warranted?" *Reprod Toxicol* 22:4 (2006): 688–693.

81. National Center for Complementary and Alternative Medicine. "Herbs at a Glance: Feverfew." Bethesda, MD: National Center for Complementary and Alternative Medicine, National Institutes of Health, December 2006. Available online at: http://nccam.nih.gov/health/feverfew.

82. Agosti, R., R.K. Duke, J.E. Chrubasik, et al. "Effectiveness of *Petasites hybridus* Preparations in the Prophylaxis of Migraine: A Systematic Review." *Phytomedicine* 13:9–10 (2006): 743–746.

83. Grossman, W., and H. Schmidramsl. "An Extract of *Petasites hybridus* is Effective in the Prophylaxis of Migraine." *Altern Med Rev* 6:3 (2001): 303–310.

84. Diener, H.C., V.W. Rahlfs, U. Danesch. "The First Placebo-controlled Trial of a Special Butterbur Root Extract for the Prevention of Migraine: Reanalysis of Efficacy Criteria." *Eur Neurol* 51:2 (2004): 89–97.

85. Lipton. R.B., H. Göbel, K.M. Einhäupl, et al. "*Petasites hybridus* Root (Butterbur) Is an Effective Preventive Treatment for Migraine." *Neurology* 63:12 (2004): 2240–2244.

86. Pothmann, R., and U. Danesch. "Migraine Prevention in Children and Adolescents: Results of an Open Study with a Special Butterbur Root Extract." *Headache* 45:3 (2005): 196–203.

Chapter 6: Supportive Nutrition

1. Brower, V. "Ancient Herb Suppresses Inflammation." *Life Extension Magazine* (March 2007).

2. Topol, E.J. "Failing the Public Health—Rofecoxib, Merck, and the FDA." *N Engl J Med* 351:17 (2004): 1707–1709.

3. Bertolini, A., A. Ottani, M. Sandrini. "Selective COX-2 Inhibitors and Dual Acting Anti-inflammatory Drugs: Critical Remarks." *Curr Med Chem* 9:10 (2002): 1033–1043.

4. Srivastava, R., and R.C. Srimal. "Modification of Certain Inflammation-induced Biochemical Changes by Curcumin." *Indian J Med Res* 81 (1985): 215–223.

5. Stix, G. "Spice Healer." *Sci Am* (January 2007).

6. Kutluay, S.B., J. Doroghazi, M.E. Roemer, et al. "Curcumin Inhibits Herpes Simplex Virus Immediate-early Gene Expression by a Mechanism Independent of p300/CBP Histone Acetyltransferase Activity." *Virology* 373:2 (2008): 239–247. Bourne, K.Z., N. Bourne, S.F. Reising, et al. "Plant Products as Topical Microbicide Candidates: Assessment of in Vitro and in Vivo Activity Against Herpes Simplex Virus Type 2." *Antiviral Res* 42:3 (1999): 219–226.

7. Aggarwal, B.B., C. Sundaram, N. Malani, et al. "Curcumin: The Indian Solid Gold." *Adv Exp Med Biol* 595 (2007): 1–75.

8. Satoskar, R.R., S.J. Shah, S.G. Shenoy. "Evaluation of Anti-inflammatory Property of Curcumin (Diferuloyl Methane) in Patients with Postoperative Inflammation." *Int J Clin Pharmacol Ther Toxicol* 24 (1986): 651–654. Lal, B., A.K. Kapoor, P.K. Agrawal, et al. "Role of Curcumin in Idiopathic Inflammatory Orbital Pseudotumours." *Phytother Res* 14 (2000): 443–447.

9. Yang, F., G.P. Lim, A.N. Begum, et al. "Curcumin Inhibits Formation of Amyloid Beta Oligomers and Fibrils, Binds Plaques, and Reduces Amyloid in Vivo." *J Biol Chem* 280:7 (2005): 5892–5901.

10. Choi, H., Y.S. Chun, S.W. Kim, et al. "Curcumin Inhibits Hypoxia-inducible Factor-1 by Degrading Aryl Hydrocarbon Receptor Nuclear Translocator: A Mechanism of Tumor Growth Inhibition." *Mol Pharmacol* 70:5 (2006): 1664–1671. Aggarwla, B.B., and S. Shishodia. "Molecular Targets of Dietary Agents for Prevention and Therapy of Cancer." *Biochem Pharmacol* 71:10 (2006): 1397–1421.

11. Marotta, F., Y.R. Shield, T. Bamba, et al. "Hepatoprotective Effect of a Curcumin/Absinthium Compound in Experimental Severe Liver Injury." *Chin J Digest Dis* 4:3 (2003): 122–127.

12. Begum, A.N., M.R. Jones, G.P. Lim, et al. "Curcumin Structure-function, Bioavailability, and Efficacy in Models of Neuroinflammation and Alzheimer's Disease." *J Pharmacol Exp Ther* 326:1 (2008): 196–208.

13. Shukla, P.K., V.K. Khanna, M.Y. Khan, et al. "Protective Effect of Curcumin against Lead Neurotoxicity in Rat." *Hum Exp Toxicol* 22:12 (2003): 653–658.

14. Shukla, P.K., V.K. Khanna, M.M. Ali, et al. "Anti-ischemic Effect of Curcumin in Rat Brain." *Neurochem Res* 33:6 (2008): 1036–1043.

15. Rao, C.V. "Regulation of COX and LOX by Curcumin." *Adv Exp Med Biol* 595 (2007): 213–226.

16. Kawanishi, S., S. Oikawa, M. Murata. "Evaluation for Safety of Antioxidant Chemopreventive Agents." *Antioxid Redox Signal* 7:11–12 (2005): 1728–1739.

17. Hickey, S., and H. Roberts. *Ascorbate: The Science of Vitamin C.* Morrisville, NH: Lulu Press, 2004.

18. Anand, P., A.B. Kunnumakkara, R.A. Newman et al. "Bioavailability of Curcumin: Problems and Promises." *Mol Pharm* 4:6 (2007): 807–818.

19. Shoba, G., D. Joy, T. Joseph, et al. "Influence of Piperine on the Pharmacokinetics of Curcumin in Animals and Human Volunteers." *Planta Med* 64:4 (1998): 353–356.

20. Bano, G., R.K. Raina, U. Zutshi, et al. "Effect of Piperine on Bioavailability and Pharmacokinetics of Propranolol and Theophylline in Healthy Volunteers." *Eur J Clin Pharm* 41:6 (1991): 615–617.

21. Kiefer, D. "Novel Turmeric Compound Delivers Much More Curcumin to the Blood." *Life Extension Magazine* (October 2007).

22. Bisht, S., G. Feldmann, S. Soni, et al. "Polymeric Nanoparticle-encapsulated Curcumin ("Nanocurcumin"): A Novel Strategy for Human Cancer Therapy." *J Nanobiotechnol* 5 (2007): 3.

23. Bhatnagar, D., and P.N. Durrington. "Omega-3 Fatty Acids: Their Role in the Prevention and Treatment of Atherosclerosis-related Risk Factors and Complications." *Int J Clin Pract* 57:4 (2003): 305–314.

24. Harel, Z., G. Gascon, S. Riggs, et al. "Supplementation with Omega-3 Polyunsaturated Fatty Acids in the Management of Recurrent Migraines in Adolescents." *J Adolesc Health* 31:2 (2002): 154–161.

25. Tripoli, E., M. Giammanco, G. Tabacchi, et al. "The Phenolic Compounds of Olive Oil: Structure, Biological Activity and Beneficial Effects on Human Health." *Nutr Res Rev* 18 (2005): 98–112.

26. Beauchamp, G.K., R.S.J. Keast, D. Morel, et al. "Phytochemistry: Ibuprofen-like Activity in Extra-virgin Olive Oil." *Nature* 437 (2005): 45–46.

27. Pradalier, A., P. Bakouche, G. Baudesson, et al. "Failure of Omega-3 Polyunsaturated Fatty Acids in Prevention of Migraine: A Double-blind Study versus Placebo." *Cephalalgia* 21:8 (2001): 818–822.

28. McCarty, M.F. "Magnesium Taurate and Fish Oil for Prevention of Migraine." *Med Hypotheses* 47:6 (1996): 461–466.

29. Gerhardt, H., F. Seifert, P. Buvari, et al. "Therapy of Active Crohn Disease with *Boswellia serrata* Extract H 15." *Z Gastroenterol* 39:1 (2001): 11–17.

30. Gupta, I., A. Parihar, P. Malhotra, et al. "Effects of Gum Resin of *Boswellia serrata* in Patients with Chronic Colitis." *Planta Med* 67:5 (2001): 391–395.

31. Shao, Y., C.T. Ho, C.K. Chin, et al. "Inhibitory Activity of Boswellic Acids from *Boswellia serrata* against Human Leukemia HL-60 Cells in Culture." *Planta Med* 64:4 (1998): 328–331.

32. Sengupta, K., K.V. Alluri, A.R. Satish, et al. "A Double-blind, Randomized, Placebo-controlled Study of the Efficacy and Safety of 5-Loxin® for Treatment

of Osteoarthritis of the Knee." *Arth Res Ther* 10 (2008): R85. Poff, C.D., and M. Balazy. "Drugs that Target Lipoxygenases and Leukotrienes as Emerging Therapies for Asthma and Cancer." *Curr Drug Targets Inflamm Allergy* 3:1 (2004): 19–33.

33. Safayhi. H., T. Mack, J. Sabieraj, et al. "Boswellic Acids: Novel, Specific, Nonredox Inhibitors of 5-Lipoxygenase." *J Pharmacol Exp Ther* 261:3 (1992): 1143–1146.

34. Russell, A.L., and M.F. McCarty. "Glucosamine for Migraine Prophylaxis?" *Med Hypotheses* 55:3 (2000): 195–198.

35. Drewyer, G.E. "Chondroitin for Migraine." *J Michigan State Med Soc* 39 (1941): 486; reported in *J Nerv Mental Dis* 94:2 (1941): 233.

36. Fusco, B.M., S. Marabini, C.A. Maggi, et al. "Preventative Effect of Repeated Nasal Applications of Capsaicin in Cluster Headache." *Pain* 59:3 (1994): 321–325.

37. Perry, W. "A Pepper A Day Keeps The Migraines Away!" Press release, Free-Press-Release.com, November 24, 2004.

38. Shaw, K., J. Turner, C. Del Mar. "Tryptophan and 5-Hydroxytryptophan for Depression." *Cochrane Database Syst Rev* 1 (2002): CD003198.

39. Sicuteri, F. "The Ingestion of Serotonin Precursors (L-5-Hydroxytryptophan and L-Tryptophan) Improves Migraine Headache." *Headache* 13:1 (1973): 19–22. Longo, G., I. Rudoi. M. Iannuccelli, et al. "Treatment of Essential Headache in Developmental Age with L-5-HTP (Cross-over Double-blind Study versus Placebo)." *Pediatr Med Chir* 6:2 (1984): 241–245.

40. Nagata, E., M. Shibata, J. Hamada, et al. "Plasma 5-Hydroxytryptamine (5-HT) in Migraine During an Attack-Free Period." *Headache* 46:4 (2006): 592–596.

41. Maissen, C.P., and H.P. Ludin. "Comparison of the Effect of 5-Hydroxytryptophan and Propranolol in the Interval Treatment of Migraine." *Schweiz Med Wochenschr* 121:43 (1991): 1585–1590.

42. Titus, F., A. Dávalos, J. Alom, et al. "5-Hydroxytryptophan versus Methysergide in the Prophylaxis of Migraine: Randomized Clinical Trial." *Eur Neurol* 25:5 (1986): 327–329.

43. De Benedittis, G., and R. Massei. "Serotonin Precursors in Chronic Primary Headache: A Double-blind Cross-over Study with L-5-Hydroxytryptophan vs. Placebo." *J Neurosurg Sci* 29:3 (1985): 239–248.

44. Turner, E.H., and A.D. Blackwell. "5-Hydroxytryptophan Plus SSRIs for Interferon-induced Depression: Synergistic Mechanisms for Normalizing Synaptic Serotonin." *Med Hypotheses* 65 (2005): 138–144.

45. Croonenberghs, J., R. Verkerk, S. Scharpe, et al. "Serotonergic Disturbances in Autistic Disorder: L-5-Hydroxytryptophan Administration to

Autistic Youngsters Increases the Blood Concentrations of Serotonin in Patients but Not in Controls." *Life Sci* 76:19 (2005): 2171–2183.

46. Croonenberghs, J., L. Delmeire, R. Verkerk, et al. "Peripheral Markers of Serotonergic and Noradrenergic Function in Post-pubertal, Caucasian Males with Autistic Disorder." *Neuropsychopharmacology* 22:3 (2000): 275–283.

47. Lin, J.N. "Overview of Migraine." *J Neurosci Nursing* 33:1 (2001): 6–13.

48. Wiedermann, U., X.J. Chen, L. Enerback, et al. "Vitamin A Deficiency Increases Inflammatory Responses, Basic Immunology." *Scand J Immunol* 44:6 (1996): 578–584. Reifen, R. "Vitamin A as an Anti-inflammatory Agent." *Proc Nutr Soc* 61:3 (2002): 397–400.

49. Braaf, M.M. (1951) "Migraine Headache: An Analysis of 124 Cases Treated by Head-traction Manipulation and Thiamin Chloride." *N Y State J Med* 31:4 (1951): 528–533. Braaf, M.M. "Migraine Headache Treated Successfully by Head-traction Manipulation and Thiamin Chloride." *N Y State J Med* 49:15 (1949): 1812–1816.

50. Panetta, J., L.J. Smith, A.J. Boneh. "Effect of High-dose Vitamins, Coenzyme Q and High-fat Diet in Paediatric Patients with Mitochondrial Diseases." *Inherit Metab Dis* 27:4 (2004): 487–498.

51. Malouf, R., and J. Grimley Evans. "The Effect of Vitamin B_6 on Cognition." *Cochrane Database Syst Rev* 4 (2003): CD004393.

52. Gaby, A.R. "Natural Approaches to Epilepsy." *Altern Med Rev* 12:1 (2007): 9–24.

53. Kleijnen, J., G. Ter Riet, P. Knipschild. "Vitamin B_6 in the Treatment of the Premenstrual Syndrome—A Review." *Br J Obstet Gynaecol* 97:9 (1990): 847–852.

54. Williams, A.L., A. Cotter, A. Sabina, et al. "The Role for Vitamin B_6 as Treatment for Depression: A Systematic Review." *Fam Pract* 22:5 (2005): 532–537.

55. Vutyavanich, T., S. Wongtra-ngan, R. Ruangsri. "Pyridoxine for Nausea and Vomiting of Pregnancy: A Randomized, Double-blind, Placebo-controlled Trial." *Am J Obstet Gynecol* 173:3 Part 1 (1995): 881–884.

56. Bender, D.A. "Non-nutritional Uses of Vitamin B_6." *Br J Nutr* 81:1 (1999): 7–20.

57. Food and Nutrition Board. "Biotin." In *Dietary Reference Intakes: Thiamin, Riboflavin, Niacin, Vitamin B_6, Vitamin B_{12}, Pantothenic Acid, Biotin, and Choline.* Washington, DC: National Academy Press, 1998.

58. Frosst, P., H.J. Blom, R. Milos, et al. "A Candidate Genetic Risk Factor for Vascular Disease: A Common Mutation in Methylenetetrahydrofolate Reductase." *Nat Genet* 10 (1995): 111–113. Weisberg, I., P. Tran, B. Christensen, et al. "A Second Genetic Polymorphism in Methylenetetrahydrofolate Reductase

(MTHFR) Associated with Decreased Enzyme Activity." *Mol Genet Metab* 64 (1998): 169–172.

59. Ferraris, E., N. Marzocchi, D. Brovia, et al. "Homocysteine Levels and Cardiovascular Disease in Migraine with Aura." *Headache* 4:2 (2003): 62–66. Moat, S.J., D. Lang, I.F. McDowell, et al. "Folate Homocysteine, Endothelial Function and Cardiovascular Disease." *J Nutr Biochem* 15:2 (2004): 64–79.

60. Di Rosa, G., S. Attinà, M. Spanò, et al. "Efficacy of Folic Acid in Children with Migraine, Hyperhomocysteinemia and MTHFR Polymorphisms." *Headache* 47:9 (2007): 1342–1344.

61. Hickey, S., H.J. Roberts, R.F. Cathcart. "Dynamic Flow." *J Orthomolecular Med* 20:4 (2005): 237–244.

62. Hickey, S., and H. Roberts. *Ascorbate: The Science of Vitamin C.* Morrisville, NH: Lulu Press, 2004.

63. Hickey, S., and A. Saul. *Vitamin C: The Real Story.* Laguna Beach, CA: Basic Health Publications, 2008.

64. Holick, M.F., and T.C. Chen. "Vitamin D Deficiency: A Worldwide Problem with Health Consequences." *Am J Clin Nutr* 87:4 (2008): 1080S–1086S.

65. Thys-Jacobs, S. "Alleviation of Migraines with Therapeutic Vitamin D and Calcium." *Headache* 34:10 (1994): 590–592.

66. Hardwick, L.L., M.R. Jones, N. Brautbar, et al. "Magnesium Absorption: Mechanisms and the Influence of Vitamin D, Calcium and Phosphate." *J Nutr* 121:1 (1991): 13–23.

67. Murphy, T.H., R.L. Schnaar, J.T. Coyle. "Immature Cortical Neurons are Uniquely Sensitive to Glutamate Toxicity by Inhibition of Cystine Uptake." *FASEB J* 4:6 (1990): 1624–1633.

68. Stuttaford, T. "Is My High-powered New Job Making My Migraine Worse?" *The Times of London* (December 8, 2005).

69. Fragoso, Y.D. "Reduction of Migraine Attacks during the Use of Warfarin." *Headache* 37:10 (1997): 667–668.

70. Kowacs, P.A., E.J. Piovesan, R.W. de Campos, et al. "Warfarin as a Therapeutic Option in the Control of Chronic Cluster Headache: A Report of Three Cases." *J Headache Pain* 6:5 (2005): 417–419.

71. Suresh, C.G., D. Neal, M.O. Coupe. "Warfarin Treatment and Migraine." *Postgrad Med J* 70:819 (1994): 37–38.

72. Rahimtoola, H., A.C. Egberts, H. Buurma, et al. "Reduction in the Intensity of Abortive Migraine Drug Use during Coumarin Therapy." *Headache* 41:8 (2001): 768–773.

73. Wammes-van der Heijden, E.A., C.C. Tijssen, A.R. van't Hoff, et al. "A Thromboembolic Predisposition and the Effect of Anticoagulants on Migraine." *Headache* 44:5 (2004): 399–402.

74. Kiechl, S., J. Schwaiger, H. Stockner, et al. "Burden of Atherosclerosis and Risk of Venous Thromboembolism in Migraine Patients." *Cerebrovasc Dis* 25:Suppl 2 (2008): 63.

75. McCarty, M.F. "Magnesium Taurate and Fish Oil for Prevention of Migraine." *Med Hypotheses* 47:6 (1996): 461–466.

76. Ibid.

77. Rothrock, J.F., K.R. Mar, T.L. Yaksh, et al. "Cerebrospinal Fluid Analyses in Migraine Patients and Controls." *Cephalalgia* 15:6 (1995): 489–493.

78. Martínez, F., J. Castillo, R. Leira, et al. "Taurine Levels in Plasma and Cerebrospinal Fluid in Migraine Patients." *Headache* 33:6 (2005): 324–327.

79. Junyent, F., J. Utrera, R. Romero, et al. "Prevention of Epilepsy by Taurine Treatments in Mice Experimental Model." *J Neurosci Res* 87:6 (2009): 1500–1508.

80. Kirchner, A., J. Breustedt, B. Rosche, et al. "Effects of Taurine and Glycine on Epileptiform Activity Induced by Removal of Mg^{2+} in Combined Rat Entorhinal Cortex-Hippocampal Slices." *Epilepsia* 44:9 (2003): 1145–1152.

81. El Idrissi, A., J. Messing, J. Scalia, et al. "Prevention of Epileptic Seizures by Taurine." *Adv Exp Med Biol* 526 (2003): 515–525.

82. Birdsall, T.C. "Therapeutic Applications of Taurine." *Altern Med Rev* 3:2 (1998): 128–136.

83. Chayasirisobhon, S. "Use of a Pine Bark Extract and Antioxidant Vitamin Combination Product as Therapy for Migraine in Patients Refractory to Pharmacologic Medication." *Headache* 46:5 (2006): 788–793.

84. Bain, B. "Benefits of *Ginkgo biloba*." *Br Med J* 328:7447 (2004): 1072. Yarnell, E., and K. Abascal. "Botanical Medicines for Headache." *Altern Complement Ther* 13:3 (2007): 148–152.

85. Burke, B.E., R.D. Olson, B.J. Cusack. "Randomized, Controlled Trial of Phytoestrogen in the Prophylactic Treatment of Menstrual Migraine." *Biomed Pharmacother* 56:6 (2002): 283–288. Ferrante, F., E. Fusco, P. Calabresi, et al. "Phyto-oestrogens in the Prophylaxis of Menstrual Migraine." *Clin Neuropharmacol* 27:3 (2004): 137–140.

86. Mathes, R.W., K.E. Malone, J.R. Daling, et al. "Migraine in Postmenopausal Women and the Risk of Invasive Breast Cancer." *Cancer Epidemiol Biomarkers Prev* 17 (2008): 3116–3122.

87. Maizels, M., A. Blumenfeld, R. Burchette. "A Combination of Riboflavin, Magnesium, and Feverfew for Migraine Prophylaxis: A Randomized Trial." *Headache* 44:9 (2004): 885–890.

88. Shrivastava, R., J.C. Pechadre, G.W. John. "*Tanacetum parthenium* and *Salix alba* (Mig-RL) Combination in Migraine Prophylaxis: A Prospective, Open-label Study." *Clin Drug Investig* 26:5 (2006): 287–296.

Chapter 7: Stopping an Attack

1. MaassenVanDenBrink, A., M. Reekers, W.A. Bax, et al. "Coronary Side-effect Potential of Current and Prospective Anti-migraine Drugs." *Circulation* 98 (1998): 25–30.

2. Visser, W.H., R.H.M. de Vriend, N.M. Jaspers, et al. "Sumatriptan in Clinical Practice: A 2-year Review of 453 Migraine Patients." *Neurology* 47 (1996): 46–51.

3. Limmroth, V., et al. "Headache after Frequent Use of Serotonin Agonists Zolmitriptan and Naratriptan." *Lancet* 353 (1999): 378.

4. British Association for the Study of Headache. "Guidelines for All Doctors in the Diagnosis and Management of Migraine and Tension-type Headache." London: British Association for the Study of Headache, 2004.

5. Buckner, K.D., M.L. Chavez, E.C. Raney, et al. "Health Food Stores' Recommendations for Nausea and Migraines During Pregnancy." *Ann Pharmacother* 39:2 (2005): 274–279.

6. Hoffman, T. "Ginger: An Ancient Remedy and Modern Miracle Drug." *Hawaii Med J* 66:12 (2007): 326–327. Langner, E., and S. Greifenberg Gruenwald "Ginger: History and Use." *J Adv Ther* 15:1 (1998): 25–44.

7. Butters, D.E., and M.W. Whitehouse. "Treating Inflammation: Some (Needless) Difficulties for Gaining Acceptance of Effective Natural Products and Traditional Medicines." *Inflammopharmacology* 11:1 (2003): 97–110. Ojewole, J.A. "Analgesic, Anti-inflammatory and Hypoglycaemic Effects of Ethanol Extract of *Zingiber officinale* (Roscoe) Rhizomes (Zingiberaceae) in Mice and Rats." *Phytother Res* 20:9 (2006): 764–772. Zhou, H.L., Y.M. Deng, Q.M. Xie. "The Modulatory Effects of the Volatile Oil of Ginger on the Cellular Immune Response in Vitro and in Vivo in Mice." *J Ethnopharmacol* 105:1-2 (2006): 301–305. Grzanna, R., L. Lindmark, C.G. Frondoza. "Ginger—An Herbal Medicinal Product with Broad Anti-inflammatory Actions." *J Med Food* 8:2 (2005): 125–132.

8. Singh, G., I.P. Kapoor, P. Singh, et al. "Chemistry, Antioxidant and Antimicrobial Investigations on Essential Oil and Oleoresins of *Zingiber officinale*." *Food Chem Toxicol* 46:10 (2008): 3295–3302. Ali, B.H., G. Blunden, M.O. Tanira, et al. "Some Phytochemical, Pharmacological and Toxicological Properties of Ginger (*Zingiber officinale* Roscoe): A Review of Recent Research." *Food Chem Toxicol* 46:2 (2008): 409–420.

9. Mustafa, T., and K.C. Srivastava. "Ginger (*Zingiber officinale*) in Migraine Headache." *J Ethnopharmacol* 29:3 (1990): 267–273.

10. Miller, L.G. "Herbal Medicinals: Selected Clinical Considerations Focusing on Known or Potential Drug-Herb Interactions." *Arch Intern Med* 158:20 (1998): 2200–2211.

11. Buckner, K.D., M.L. Chavez, E.C. Raney, et al. "Health Food Stores' Rec-

ommendations for Nausea and Migraines During Pregnancy." *Ann Pharmacother* 39:2 (2005): 274–279.

12. Mills, E., J. Prousky, G. Raskin, et al. "The Safety of Over-the-counter Niacin: A Randomized Placebo-controlled Trial." *BMC Clin Pharmacol* 3 (2003): 4.

13. Velling, D.A., D.W. Dodick, J.J. Muir. "Sustained-release Niacin for Prevention of Migraine Headache." *Mayo Clin Proc* 78:6 (2003): 770–771.

14. Hendler, S.S. *The Doctors' Vitamin and Mineral Encyclopedia.* New York: Simon and Schuster, 1990.

15. Gedye, A. "Hypothesized Treatment for Migraines Using Low Doses of Tryptophan, Niacin, Calcium, Caffeine, and Acetylsalicylic Acid." *Med Hypotheses* 56 (2001): 91–94.

16. Prousky, J., and D. Seely. "The Treatment of Migraines and Tension-type Headaches with Intravenous and Oral Niacin (Nicotinic Acid): Systematic Review of the Literature." *Nutr J* 4 (2005): 3–10.

17. Atkinson, M. "Migraine Headache: Some Clinical Observations on the Vascular Mechanism and Its Control." *Ann Intern Med* 21 (1944): 990–997.

18. Goldzieher, J.W., and G.L. Popkin. "Treatment of Headaches with Intravenous Sodium Nicotinate." *JAMA* 131 (1946): 103–105.

19. Grenfell, R.F. "Treatment of Migraine with Nicotinic Acid." *Am Pract* 3 (1949): 542–544.

20. Grenfell, R.F. "Treatment of Tension Headache." *Am Pract Dig Treat* 2 (1951): 933–936.

21. Morgan, Z.R. "Nicotinic Acid Therapy in Vasoconstriction Type of Headache." *MD State Med J* 2 (1953): 377–382. Morgan, Z.R. "A Newer Method of Nicotinic Acid Therapy in Headache of the Vasoconstrictive Type." *J Am Geriatr Soc* 3 (1955): 545–551.

22. Hall, J.A. "Enhancing Niacin's Effect for Migraine." *Cortlandt Forum* (1991): 46.

23. Prousky, J.E., and E. Sykes. "Two Case Reports on the Treatment of Acute Migraine with Niacin: Its Hypothetical Mechanism of Action upon Calcitonin Gene–related Peptide and Platelets." *J Orthomolecular Med* 18:2 (2003): 108–110.

24. Food and Nutrition Board. *Dietary Reference Intakes: Thiamin, Riboflavin, Niacin, Vitamin B_6, Vitamin B_{12}, Pantothenic Acid, Biotin, and Choline.* Washington, DC: Institute of Medicine, National Academy Press, 1998.

25. Knopp, R.H. "Evaluating Niacin in Its Various Forms." *Am J Cardiol* 86:12A (2000): 51L–56L.

26. Food and Nutrition Board. *Dietary Reference Intakes: Thiamin, Riboflavin, Niacin, Vitamin B_6, Vitamin B_{12}, Pantothenic Acid, Biotin, and Choline.* Washington, DC: Institute of Medicine, National Academy Press, 1998.

27. Christiansen, I., L.L. Thomsen, D. Daugaard, et al. "Glyceryl Trinitrate Induces Attacks of Migraine without Aura in Sufferers of Migraine with Aura." *Cephalalgia* 19:7 (1999): 660–667.

28. Olesen, J., H.K. Iversen, L.L. Thomsen. "Nitric Oxide Supersensitivity: A Possible Molecular Mechanism of Migraine Pain." *Neuroreport* 4:8 (1993): 1027–1030. Olesen, J., L.L. Thomsen, H. Iversen. "Nitric Oxide is a Key Molecule in Migraine and Other Vascular Headaches." *Trends Pharmacol Sci* 15:5 (1994): 149–153.

29. Anonymous. "Vitamin B_{12} Therapy of Headache." *Tidsskr Nor Laegeforen* 71:12 (1951): 398. Dalsgaard-Nielsen, T. "Vitamin B_{12} in Therapy of Migraine and Psychogenic Headache." *Ugeskr Laeger* 114:34 (1952): 1143–1144. Sicuteri, F., and U. Becattini. "Effect of Vitamin B_{12} on Medical Headaches; Observations and Critical Notes." *Minerva Med* 50:8 (1959): 197–204.

30. van der Kuy, P.H., F.W. Merkus, J.J. Lohman, et al. "Hydroxocobalamin, a Nitric Oxide Scavenger, in the Prophylaxis of Migraine: An Open, Pilot Study." *Cephalalgia* 22:7 (2002): 513–519.

31. Hutto, B.R. "Folate and Cobalamin in Psychiatric Illness." *Compr Psychiatry* 38:6 (1997): 305–314. Penninx, B.W., J.M. Guralnik, L. Ferrucci, et al. "Vitamin B($_{12}$) Deficiency and Depression in Physically Disabled Older Women: Epidemiologic Evidence from the Women's Health and Aging Study." *Am J Psychiatry* 157:5 (2000): 715–721. Tiemeier, H., H.R. van Tuijl, A. Hofman, et al. "Vitamin B_{12}, Folate, and Homocysteine in Depression: The Rotterdam Study." *Am J Psychiatry* 159:12 (2002): 2099–2101.

32. Cady, R.K., C.P. Schreiber, M.E. Beach, et al. "Gelstat Migraine (Sublingually Administered Feverfew and Ginger Compound) for Acute Treatment of Migraine When Administered During the Mild Pain Phase." *Med Sci Monit* 11:9 (2005): PI65–PI69.

33. Mauskop, A., and B.M. Altura. "Role of Magnesium in the Pathogenesis and Treatment of Migraines." *Clin Neurosci* 5:1 (1998): 24–27. Mauskop, A., B.T. Altura, R.Q. Cracco, et al. "Intravenous Magnesium Sulfate Rapidly Alleviates Headaches of Various Types." *Headache* 36:3 (1996): 154–160.

34. Ibid.

35. Demirkaya, S., O. Vural, B. Dora, et al. "Efficacy of Intravenous Magnesium Sulfate in the Treatment of Acute Migraine Attacks." *Headache* 41:2 (2001): 171–177.

36. Mauskop, A., B.T. Altura, R.Q. Cracco, et al. "Intravenous Magnesium Sulphate Relieves Migraine Attacks in Patients with Low Serum Ionized Magnesium Levels: A Pilot Study." *Clin Sci* 89 (1995): 633–636.

Chapter 8: Physical Therapies for Migraines

1. Vijayan, N. "Head Band for Migraine Headache Relief." *Headache* 33:1 (1993): 40–42.

2. Landy, S.H., and B. Griffin. "Pressure, Heat, and Cold Help Relieve Headache Pain." *Arch Fam Med* 9:9 (2000): 792–793.

3. Singh, R.K., A. Martinez, P. Baxter. "Head Cooling for Exercise-induced Headache." *J Child Neurol* 21:12 (2006): 1067–1068.

4. Robbins, L.D. "Cryotherapy for Headache." *Headache* 29:9 (1989): 598–600.

5. Diamond, S., and F.G. Freitag. "Cold as an Adjunctive Therapy for Headache." *Postgrad Med* 79:1 (1986): 305–309.

6. Lance, J.W. "The Controlled Application of Cold and Heat by a New Device (Migra-lief Apparatus) in the Treatment of Headache." *Headache* 28:7 (1988): 458–461.

7. Vijayan, N. "Head Band for Migraine Headache Relief." *Headache* 33:1 (1993): 40–42.

8. Fumal, A., V. Bohotin, M. Vandenheede, et al. "Transcranial Magnetic Stimulation in Migraine: A Review of Facts and Controversies." *Acta Neurol Belg* 103:3 (2003): 144–154.

9. Aurora, S.K., B.K. Ahmad, K.M. Welch, et al. "Transcranial Magnetic Stimulation Confirms Hyperexcitability of Occipital Cortex in Migraine." *Neurology* 50:4 (1998): 1111–1114. Aurora, S.K., and K.M. Welch. "Brain Excitability in Migraine: Evidence from Transcranial Magnetic Stimulation Studies." *Curr Opin Neurol* 11:3 (1998): 205–209.

10. Aurora, S.K., K.M. Welch, F. Al-Sayed. "The Threshold for Phosphenes is Lower in Migraine." *Cephalalgia* 23:4 (2003): 258–263.

11. Gunaydin, S., A. Soysal, T. Atay, et al. "Motor and Occipital Cortex Excitability in Migraine Patients." *Can J Neurol Sci* 33:1 (2006): 63–67.

12. Fumal, A., V. Bohotin, M. Vandenheede, et al. "Transcranial Magnetic Stimulation in Migraine: A Review of Facts and Controversies." *Acta Neurol Belg* 103:3 (2003): 144–154. Valeriani, M., B. Fierro, F. Brighina. "Brain Excitability in Migraine: Hyperexcitability or Inhibited Inhibition?" *Pain* 132:1–2 (2007): 219–220.

13. O'Reardon, J.P., J.F. Fontecha, M.A. Cristancho, et al. "Unexpected Reduction in Migraine and Psychogenic Headaches Following rTMS Treatment for Major Depression: A Report of Two Cases." *CNS Spectr* 12:12 (2007): 921–925.

14. Clarke, B.M., A.R. Upton, M.V. Kamath, et al. "Transcranial Magnetic Stimulation for Migraine: Clinical Effects." *J Headache Pain* 7:5 (2006): 341–346

15. "Magnetic Device Short-circuits Migraine Headaches, Suggests Early Research." 48th Annual Scientific Meeting of the American Headache Society press release, June 22, 2006.

16. Hickey, S., A.S. Atkins, A.K. Hairul Nizam Pengiran Haji Ali. "Mobile Technology: The Global Risk Experiment." Invited paper, APIIT SD, ICACCT, 2007, 1–7.

17. Bennett, M.H., C. French, A. Schnabel, et al. "Normobaric and Hyperbaric Oxygen Therapy for Migraine and Cluster Headache." *Cochrane Database Syst Rev* 16:3 (2008): CD005219.

18. Kudrow, L. "Response of Cluster Headache Attacks to Oxygen Inhalation." *Headache* 21:1 (1981): 1–4.

19. Atochin, D.N., I.T. Demchenko, J. Astern, et al. "Contributions of Endothelial and Neuronal Nitric Oxide Synthases to Cerebrovascular Responses to Hyperoxia." *J Cerebral Blood Flow Metab* 23 (2003): 1219–1226.

20. Myers, D.E., and R.A. Myers. "A Preliminary Report on Hyperbaric Oxygen in the Relief of Migraine Headache." *Headache* 35:4 (1995): 197–199.

21. Eftedal, O.S., S. Lydersen, G. Helde, et al. "A Randomized, Double-blind Study of the Prophylactic Effect of Hyperbaric Oxygen Therapy on Migraine." *Cephalalgia* 24:8 (2004): 639–644.

22. Ernst, E., M.H. Pittler, B. Wider, et al. "Acupuncture: Its Evidence-base Is Changing." *Am J Chin Med* 35:1 (2007): 21–25.

23. Pomeranz, B., and D. Chiu. "Naloxone Blockade of Acupuncture Analgesia: Endorphin Implicated." *Life Sci* 19:11 (1976): 1757–1762. Mayer, D.J., D.D. Price, A. Rafii. "Antagonism of Acupuncture Analgesia in Man by the Narcotic Antagonist Naloxone." *Brain Res* 121:2 (1977): 368–372.

24. Melzack, R. "Acupuncture and Pain Mechanisms." *Anaesthesist* 25:5 (1976): 204–207.

25. Melzack, R., and P.D. Wall. "On the Nature of Cutaneous Sensory Mechanisms." *Brain* 85 (1962): 331–356. Melzack, R., and P.D. Wall. "Pain Mechanisms: A New Theory." *Science* 150:699 (1965): 971–979.

26. Li, K., B. Shan, J. Xu, et al. "Changes in fMRI in the Human Brain Related to Different Durations of Manual Acupuncture Needling." *J Altern Complement Med* 12:7 (2006): 615–623. Pariente, J., P. White, R.S. Frackowiak, et al. "Expectancy and Belief Modulate the Neuronal Substrates of Pain Treated by Acupuncture." *Neuroimage* 25:4 (2005): 1161–1167.

27. Shen, J. "Research on the Neurophysiological Mechanisms of Acupuncture: Review of Selected Studies and Methodological Issues." *J Altern Complement Med* 7:Suppl 1 (2001): S121–S127.

28. Liu, J.L., X.W. Han, S.N. Su. "The Role of Frontal Neurons in Pain and Acupuncture Analgesia." *Sci China B* 33:8 (1990): 938–945.

29. Diener, H., K. Kronfeld, G. Boewing, et al.; The GERAC Migraine Study Group. "Efficacy of Acupuncture for the Prophylaxis of Migraine: A Multicentre Randomised Controlled Clinical Trial." *Lancet Neurol* 5 (2006): 310–316.

30. Dibble, S.L., J. Luce, B.A. Cooper, et al. "Acupressure for Chemotherapy-induced Nausea and Vomiting: A Randomized Clinical Trial." *Oncol Nurs Forum* 34:4 (2007): 813–820.

31. Lee, A., and M.L. Done. "Stimulation of the Wrist Acupuncture Point P6 for Preventing Postoperative Nausea and Vomiting." *Cochrane Database Syst Rev* 3 (2004): CD003281. Ezzo, J.M., M.A. Richardson, A. Vickers, et al. "Acupuncture-point Stimulation for Chemotherapy-induced Nausea or Vomiting." *Cochrane Database Syst Rev* 2 (2006): CD002285.

32. Melchart, D., K. Linde, B. Berman, et al. "Acupuncture for Idiopathic Headache." *Cochrane Database Syst Rev* 1 (2001): CD001218.

33. Ibid.

34. Tuchin, P.J., H. Pollard, R. Bonello. "A Randomized Controlled Trial of Chiropractic Spinal Manipulative Therapy for Migraine." *J Manipulative Physiol Ther* 23:2 (2000): 91–95. Tuchin, P.J. "A Twelve-month Clinical Trial of Chiropractic Spinal Manipulative Therapy for Migraine." *Australas Chiropr Osteopathy* 8:2 (1999): 61–65.

35. Upledger, J.E. "Craniosacral Therapy." *Phys Ther* 75:4 (1995): 328–330.

36. Nestoriuc, Y., A. Martin, W. Rief, et al. "Biofeedback Treatment for Headache Disorders: A Comprehensive Efficacy Review." *Appl Psychophysiol Biofeedback* 33:3 (2008): 125–140.

37. Lawler, S.P., and L.D. Cameron. "A Randomized, Controlled Trial of Massage Therapy as a Treatment for Migraine." *Ann Behav Med* 32:1 (2006): 50–59.

Chapter 9: Get Your Life Back

1. Teschke, R., and A. Wolff. "Kava Hepatotoxicity: Regulatory Data Selection and Causality Assessment." *Dig Liver Dis* (May 26, 2009). Epub ahead of print.

2. Teschke, R., A. Schwarzenboeck, A. Akinci. "Kava Hepatotoxicity: A European View." *N Z Med J* 121:1283 (2008): 90–98.

INDEX

193

ABOUT THE AUTHOR

Steve Hickey, Ph.D., received his doctorate in medical biophysics from the University of Manchester, England. He is a member of the Institute of Biology (Pharmacology), a chartered biologist, and a former member of the British Computer Society. He has published over 100 scientific publications and is the co-author of *Vitamin C: The Real Story* (Basic Health, 2009) and other books on science and health.